Acne

Proven Natural Remedies for Acne-free Skin

(Easy Natural Home Remedies for Acne & How to Prevent It)

Kirby Sanchez

Published By **Simon Dough**

Kirby Sanchez

All Rights Reserved

Acne: Proven Natural Remedies for Acne-free Skin (Easy Natural Home Remedies for Acne & How to Prevent It)

ISBN 978-1-7772550-1-5

No part of this guidebook shall be reproduced in any form without permission in writing from the publisher except in the case of brief quotations embodied in critical articles or reviews.

Legal & Disclaimer

The information contained in this book is not designed to replace or take the place of any form of medicine or professional medical advice. The information in this book has been provided for educational & entertainment purposes only.

The information contained in this book has been compiled from sources deemed reliable, and it is accurate to the best of the Author's knowledge; however, the Author cannot guarantee its accuracy and validity and cannot be held liable for any errors or omissions. Changes are periodically made to this book. You must consult your doctor or get professional medical advice before using any of the suggested remedies, techniques, or information in this book.

Upon using the information contained in this book, you agree to hold harmless the Author from and against any damages, costs, and expenses, including any legal fees potentially resulting from the application of any of the information provided by this guide. This disclaimer applies to any damages or injury caused by the use and application, whether directly or indirectly, of any advice or information presented, whether for breach of contract, tort, negligence, personal injury, criminal intent, or under any other cause of action.

You agree to accept all risks of using the information presented inside this book. You need to consult a professional medical practitioner in order to ensure you are both able and healthy enough to participate in this program.

Table Of Contents

Chapter 1: The Role of Diet and Acne 1

Chapter 2: Skincare Routines 16

Chapter 3: Natural Remedies for Acne ... 39

Chapter 4: The Importance of Lifestyle In Acne Prevention 57

Chapter 5: Medical Treatments for Acne 74

Chapter 6: Preventing Acne Scars and Treating Existing Scars 100

Chapter 7: Understanding Acne 113

Chapter 8: Acne in Maturity 173

Chapter 9: My Zits 179

Chapter 1: The Role of Diet and Acne

The Connection between Diet and Acne

While the relationship among weight-reduction plan and pimples has been a subject of debate for decades, current studies suggests that sure nutritional elements can make a contribution to the development or exacerbation of acne. In this bankruptcy, we are able to explore the connection among weight loss program and zits, discussing specific meals and vitamins that may impact your pores and pores and skin's health and providing dietary tips. While weight loss program is surely one problem inside the development of pimples, making aware meals alternatives and preserving a balanced, nutrient-rich weight loss program can make a contribution to improved pores and skin health. Keep in mind that man or woman responses to dietary changes also can range, and what works for one man or woman might not work for some different. Experiment with unique dietary adjustments, and be aware about how your pores and pores and pores and skin reacts to find out which changes may be maximum useful for you. If you are uncertain approximately making nutritional changes or suspect that you could have a nutrient deficiency, consult a healthcare expert or registered dietitian for custom designed advice.

Foods to Avoid:

While man or woman reactions to food can also moreover variety, fine components and components have been associated with pimples improvement or exacerbation. Here is a listing of substances and food agencies that you may need to bear in mind keeping off or restricting when you have zits-prone pores and pores and skin:

1. High-glycemic carbohydrates: Foods with a immoderate glycemic index can purpose speedy spikes in blood sugar and

insulin ranges, likely principal to stepped forward sebum production and clogged pores. Examples of immoderate-glycemic factors embody:

White bread

White rice

Sugary cereals

Cookies and desserts

Potato chips

2. Dairy products: Some research has encouraged a link among dairy consumption and zits, especially with skim milk. If you watched that dairy can be contributing on your zits, go through in mind lowering your consumption of:

Milk (particularly skim milk)

Cheese

Ice cream

Yogurt

three. Sugary and processed food: Foods immoderate in sugar and horrific fats can purpose infection, disrupt hormonal stability, and shortage essential vitamins for healthful pores and skin. Limit your consumption of:

Candy and chocolate (particularly milk chocolate)

Soda and sugary liquids

Processed snack food (e.G., chips, crackers, and pastries)

Fast food

four. Refined and hydrogenated oils: Consuming massive quantities of delicate and hydrogenated oils can make a contribution to contamination and an imbalance of omega-6 to omega-three fatty acids, which can also worsen acne. Limit your consumption of:

Margarine

Shortening

Processed vegetable oils (e.G., soybean, corn, and sunflower oil)

five. Alcohol and caffeine: Excessive consumption of alcohol and caffeine can make contributions to dehydration and hormonal imbalances, probably exacerbating pimples. Limit your intake of:

Alcoholic drinks

Coffee

Energy beverages

Tea (mainly if immoderate in caffeine)

6. Food allergens and sensitivities: Some human beings may also experience acne flare-u.S.A.Because of meals hypersensitive reactions or sensitivities. Common culprits embody gluten, soy, and shellfish. If you suspect a meals sensitivity or allergy,

searching for advice from a healthcare expert for steering on identifying and eliminating capacity triggers from your weight loss program.

Foods to Embrace for Acne-Prone Skin

A balanced, nutrient-wealthy food plan can contribute to more wholesome pores and skin and can help manipulate zits signs and symptoms and signs and symptoms. Here are a few components and food agencies that you need to consider embracing for clearer, greater wholesome pores and pores and skin:

1. Low-glycemic carbohydrates: Foods with a low glycemic index provide a steadier launch of power and may assist control blood sugar and insulin degrees, which can be useful for pimples-inclined pores and skin. Examples of low-glycemic ingredients embody:

Whole grains (e.G., brown rice, quinoa, whole wheat bread)

Legumes (e.G., lentils, chickpeas, black beans)

Non-starchy greens (e.G., leafy veggies, broccoli, cauliflower)

2. Omega-three fatty acids: Omega-three fatty acids have anti inflammatory homes and might assist stability the ratio of omega-6 to omega-three fatty acids, probable reducing acne symptoms and signs and symptoms. Include greater omega-three-rich substances to your diet regime, which consist of:

Fatty fish (e.G., salmon, mackerel, sardines)

Walnuts

Chia seeds

Flaxseeds

Hemp seeds

3. Antioxidant-wealthy give up end result and greens: Fruits and greens are

filled with vitamins, minerals, and antioxidants that guide wholesome pores and skin. Focus on consuming a whole lot of colorful fruits and greens, which include:

Berries (e.G., blueberries, strawberries, raspberries)

Leafy veggies (e.G., spinach, kale, Swiss chard)

Orange and yellow veggies (e.G., carrots, candy potatoes, bell peppers)

Cruciferous vegetables (e.G., broccoli, cauliflower, Brussels sprouts)

four. Lean protein assets: Protein is vital for pores and pores and skin repair and the formation of latest pores and pores and pores and skin cells. Opt for lean sources of protein, which also can assist hold balanced blood sugar ranges:

Chicken or turkey breast

Fish

Eggs

Tofu or tempeh

Legumes (e.G., lentils, chickpeas, black beans)

five. Healthy fats: Consuming wholesome fat can help hold your pores and pores and skin moisturized and might reduce contamination. Include greater healthy fat property to your food plan, inclusive of:

Avocado

Nuts (e.G., almonds, walnuts, pistachios)

Seeds (e.G., chia seeds, flaxseeds, pumpkin seeds)

Olive oil or avocado oil

6. Probiotics: Probiotics can help aid a healthy intestine, which might also make a contribution to clearer pores and pores and skin thru decreasing contamination and enhancing nutrient absorption. Include

probiotic-rich food on your healthy eating plan, which encompass:

Greek yogurt or kefir (if dairy is not an problem for you)

Fermented foods (e.G., sauerkraut, kimchi, miso, tempeh)

7. Hydration: Drinking enough water is critical for healthful pores and pores and skin, because it permits flush pollutants from the body and permits pores and skin cell turnover. Make positive to stay well hydrated at some degree within the day through:

Drinking water

Eating water-rich stop result and greens (e.G., cucumber, watermelon, oranges)

Supplements for Clear Skin

While a balanced diet need to offer most of the vitamins critical for healthful skin, a few people may additionally advantage from taking nutritional supplements to deal with deficiencies or assist particular additives of pores and pores and skin fitness. Here are a few nutritional dietary supplements that could make contributions to clearer pores and skin:

1. Zinc: Zinc is an critical mineral that plays a crucial role in pores and pores and skin health, collectively with wound recovery, immune function, and the law of sebum production. Some studies advise that zinc supplementation might also assist reduce zits symptoms, mainly in humans with a zinc deficiency.

2. Vitamin A: Vitamin A is critical for pores and pores and skin mobile increase and differentiation, similarly to the renovation of the pores and pores and pores and skin's barrier function. Retinoids, a spinoff of weight loss plan A, are often utilized in topical acne treatments. However, oral weight-reduction plan A supplementation need to be approached

with caution, as immoderate intake can be toxic. Consult a healthcare professional earlier than beginning any nutrients A supplementation.

three. Vitamin D: Vitamin D performs a function in immune characteristic and the law of contamination, which might also effect zits development. Some research endorse that people with zits may additionally moreover moreover have decrease eating regimen D tiers. Consider getting your nutrients D ranges examined and supplementing if important, below the steerage of a healthcare expert.

four. Vitamin E: Vitamin E is an antioxidant that lets in defend the pores and skin from oxidative strain and may guide pores and skin recovery. While its feature in pimples remedy is heaps much less mounted, a few people with acne-willing pores and skin might also moreover benefit from nutrition E supplementation, in particular inside the occasion that they have got a deficiency.

5. Omega-3 fatty acids: Omega-three fatty acids have anti inflammatory homes and might assist lessen irritation associated with acne. Supplements, which encompass fish oil or algae-primarily based totally omega-three dietary dietary supplements, can assist growth your omega-three intake if you war to get enough through diet by myself.

6. Probiotics: Probiotic dietary dietary supplements can assist assist a healthy intestine microbiome, which may also make a contribution to clearer pores and pores and skin thru reducing infection and enhancing nutrient absorption. Look for a complement with quite a few strains and a high CFU (colony-forming devices) depend.

7. Niacinamide (Vitamin B3): Niacinamide has been tested to lessen contamination, adjust sebum production, and guide skin barrier function, making it a doubtlessly beneficial complement for

people with zits-inclined pores and pores and skin.

8. Biotin (Vitamin B7): Biotin is involved inside the manufacturing of keratin, a protein that makes up our skin, hair, and nails. While there may be restricted proof at the direct impact of biotin supplementation on acne, some human beings may additionally advantage from it within the occasion that they have got a biotin deficiency.

Keep in thoughts that nutritional dietary supplements need to now not replace a balanced eating regimen but can be used as an accessory to useful resource skin fitness. Before beginning any supplementation, trying to find recommendation from a healthcare professional or registered dietitian to determine which nutritional dietary dietary supplements may be suitable for you and to make certain you take the right dosages. Always follow the endorsed guidelines and be cautious of capacity interactions with medicinal tablets or unique nutritional supplements.

Chapter 2: Skincare Routines

Establishing an effective skincare ordinary is critical for dealing with acne and keeping wholesome pores and skin. This section will offer a whole guide on developing a skin care ordinary tailor-made for acne-inclined skin, masking crucial steps and issues.

Identifying Your Skin Type

Recognizing your pores and pores and skin kind is the first step to developing a customised pores and skin care routine that correctly addresses your pores and pores and skin's goals. Generally, there are four predominant pores and skin types: oily, dry, combination, and touchy. Each pores and skin kind has notable developments for you to will let you decide which magnificence your pores and pores and skin falls into:

1. Oily Skin:

Often appears shiny or greasy, specifically within the T-area (brow, nostril, and chin)

Larger, more seen pores

Prone to blackheads, whiteheads, and breakouts because of more oil production

Makeup may not final as prolonged or might also seem to "slide off" the face

To address oily pores and skin, look for oil-unfastened, non-comedogenic products that can help modify oil manufacturing without clogging pores. Ingredients like salicylic acid, niacinamide, and clay can be beneficial for shiny, zits-inclined pores and pores and pores and skin.

2. Dry Skin:

Feels tight, hard, or flaky, specially after cleansing

Smaller, less visible pores

Prone to redness, infection, and sensitivity

Makeup may additionally seem patchy or dangle to dry regions

For dry pores and pores and skin, popularity on gentle, hydrating products that assist restore moisture and shield the pores and skin's herbal barrier. Ingredients like hyaluronic acid, ceramides, and glycerin can help offer and hold moisture in the pores and skin.

3. Combination Skin:

A mixture of oily and dry areas, usually oily in the T-location and dry on the cheeks

Pore length and visibility may additionally moreover variety at some point of the face

Prone to breakouts in oily areas and dryness or flakiness in dry regions

Combination skin calls for a balanced approach, addressing every oiliness and dryness. Use mild, non-comedogenic merchandise which can assist adjust oil manufacturing in the T-sector even as imparting true sufficient hydration for the drier areas of the face.

4. Sensitive Skin:

Prone to redness, itching, stinging, or burning sensations on the same time as the use of positive merchandise

May react adversely to fragrances, dyes, or harsh elements

Can come to be effects angry or inflamed, potentially exacerbating pimples

Sensitive skin requires more care to reduce contamination and inflammation. Opt for mild, fragrance-loose, and hypoallergenic merchandise specially designed for sensitive pores and pores and skin. Patch-check new products on a small place of your skin in advance than incorporating them into your everyday to make certain they do no longer reason a reaction.

It's critical to undergo in thoughts that your pores and skin kind can alternate over the years due to factors together with age, hormones, weather, and way of life.

Periodically rethink your pores and skin kind to make sure you're using the most suitable merchandise for your modern-day wishes. If you have got were given issue figuring out your pores and pores and pores and skin kind or worries, consult a dermatologist or skin care professional for guidance.

The Importance of Cleansing

Cleansing is a vital step in any skin care habitual, serving as the inspiration for maintaining healthy, clear pores and skin. It plays a critical position in removing dust, oil, make-up, and impurities from the pores and skin's floor, preventing clogged pores and breakouts. For people with acne-prone pores and pores and skin, right cleansing is even extra essential, because it facilitates to govern more sebum production and decrease the chance of pimples flare-ups. Below are some key elements to preserve in thoughts close to the significance of cleaning for zits-willing pores and pores and pores and skin.

1. Prevents clogged pores: Acne happens whilst vain pores and pores and skin cells, oil, and specific debris collect in the pores, leading to contamination and bacterial increase. Regular cleaning permits to take away the ones impurities, keeping pores easy and decreasing the threat of breakouts.

2. Balances oil production: Cleansing can help alter oil manufacturing inside the pores and pores and skin, stopping excess sebum from contributing to zits formation. However, it is important to use a moderate purifier that doesn't strip the pores and skin of its herbal oils, as this could cause the pores and skin to deliver even more oil in response.

three. Allows for higher product absorption: Cleansing prepares the pores and skin to absorb next skin care merchandise greater effectively. By getting rid of dirt and oil, cleansers create a clean ground that lets in for better penetration of active factors for your serums, treatments, and moisturizers.

4. Reduces the hazard of infection: A buildup of impurities at the pores and pores and pores and skin can reason contamination and contamination, likely worsening pimples. Cleansing permits to get rid of those irritants, selling a calmer, greater balanced complexion.

five. Promotes wholesome pores and pores and skin cellular turnover: Regular cleansing can resource pores and skin mobile turnover by using way of way of disposing of lifeless pores and pores and skin cells and other particles from the pores and pores and skin's surface. This technique is essential for retaining a healthy, smooth complexion and stopping pimples.

6. Prevents the unfold of pimples-inflicting bacteria: Acne-inclined pores and pores and skin is frequently more susceptible to bacterial growth, which can

contribute to breakouts. Cleansing permits to take away micro organism from the skin's floor, minimizing the risk of zits flare-ups.

When cleansing zits-prone skin, it's critical to select out a gentle, non-comedogenic purifier that might not clog pores or get worse the pores and pores and pores and skin. Look for formulation specially designed for pimples-susceptible skin, containing factors like salicylic acid or benzoyl peroxide, that might help to fight acne. Additionally, avoid using harsh scrubs or brushes that would reason infection and inflammation. Cleanse your face times an afternoon – in the morning and nighttime – to hold a easy and balanced complexion. However, in case your pores and pores and skin feels too dry or indignant, you may want to adjust your cleansing normal or transfer to a gentler purifier.

Exfoliation: Types and Benefits

Exfoliation is a critical component of a pores and skin care ordinary, specially for pimples-willing pores and skin. It allows take away vain pores and skin cells, unclog pores, and promote cellular turnover, main to a smoother, clearer complexion. Regular exfoliation can enhance pores and pores and pores and skin texture, lessen the arrival of acne scars, and even assist one of a kind skincare products artwork more efficiently. In this segment, we are going to discover the two primary varieties of exfoliation and their blessings for pimples-prone pores and skin.

1. Physical Exfoliation:

Physical exfoliation includes the use of a scrub, brush, or textured material to manually get rid of useless skin cells from the skin's ground. The friction created by means of the abrasive fabric permits enhance and do away with debris, revealing brisker, greater radiant pores and skin.

Benefits of bodily exfoliation:

Instantly smoother pores and pores and skin

Improved pores and skin texture

Enhanced float and skin cell renewal

However, physical exfoliants can now and again be too harsh for zits-susceptible or sensitive pores and skin, as they may cause micro-tears, contamination, or infection. If you pick out to use a physical exfoliant, choose a slight scrub with smooth, spherical beads, or use a smooth washcloth. Be aware not to apply too much pressure and keep away from over-exfoliating, that would worsen zits.

2. Chemical Exfoliation:

Chemical exfoliants use acids or enzymes to dissolve useless pores and skin cells and sell cellular turnover. Alpha-hydroxy acids (AHAs) and beta-hydroxy acids (BHAs) are the maximum commonplace kinds of chemical exfoliants, with glycolic acid and lactic acid being well-known AHAs, and salicylic acid being a widely-used BHA.

Benefits of chemical exfoliation:

More uniform exfoliation, accomplishing deeper layers of the skin

Reduces the arrival of zits scars and hyperpigmentation

Improves pores and skin's common tone and texture

Can assist manage oil production and unclog pores

Chemical exfoliants are frequently endorsed for pimples-inclined pores and pores and pores and skin, as they will be plenty less traumatic than physical exfoliants and are extra effective at penetrating and unclogging pores. BHAs, like salicylic acid, are particularly useful for zits-prone pores and pores and pores and skin, as they are oil-soluble and might achieve deep into the pores to dissolve oil and impurities.

When incorporating exfoliation into your skincare recurring, start with a moderate product and steadily increase the frequency and intensity as your pores and pores and skin tolerates it. For maximum human beings, exfoliating 1-2 times in line with week is sufficient. Over-exfoliation can reason inflammation, dryness, and a compromised pores and pores and skin barrier, doubtlessly main to more zits. As continuously, have a observe up with a moisturizer to help keep pores and skin hydration and guard the pores and skin barrier.

Moisturizing and Hydration

Proper moisturization and hydration are important for keeping wholesome, balanced skin, even for human beings with acne-inclined pores and skin. Some human beings mistakenly bear in mind that oily or pimples-inclined pores and pores and skin does not require moisturizing, however this false impression can bring about similarly pores and pores and pores and skin issues. In truth, a lack of moisture can purpose the pores and pores and skin to overcompensate by way of way of generating extra oil, principal to improved breakouts. This section will talk the importance of moisturizing and hydration for zits-willing pores and skin and offer steerage on choosing the proper products.

1. Restoring the pores and pores and skin's barrier feature: Moisturizing lets in keep and repair the pores and skin's natural barrier, which protects it from environmental stressors, micro organism, and contamination. A wholesome pores and pores and skin barrier is crucial for preventing breakouts and selling a easy complexion.

2. Reducing inflammation and infection: Acne-susceptible pores and skin is frequently at risk of redness, irritation, and contamination. Using a moisturizer with soothing and anti inflammatory substances

(which incorporates niacinamide, aloe vera, or inexperienced tea) can assist calm the pores and skin and decrease the severity of breakouts.

three. Balancing oil production: Providing adequate hydration to the pores and pores and skin can assist regulate oil production, stopping the overproduction of sebum that could make contributions to pimples. A properly-formulated moisturizer can deliver crucial hydration with out clogging pores or exacerbating oiliness.

four. Enhancing the effectiveness of different pores and skin care merchandise: Well-moisturized pores and pores and skin is higher capable of absorb and utilize lively components in your serums, remedies, and different skin care merchandise. Maintaining right hydration can help decorate the overall effectiveness of your pores and pores and skin care ordinary.

five. Promoting pores and pores and skin recuperation: A well-hydrated, moisturized pores and pores and skin surroundings is essential for the healing method. Moisturizers can assist to assuage and restore damaged pores and pores and pores and skin, reducing the advent of acne scars and selling a smoother, extra even complexion.

When selecting a moisturizer for pimples-inclined pores and pores and pores and skin, do not forget the following tips:

Choose a lightweight, oil-loose, and non-comedogenic technique to decrease the threat of clogged pores and breakouts.

Look for additives that provide hydration with out along with oil, collectively with hyaluronic acid, glycerin, or aloe vera.

Opt for moisturizers with delivered benefits, which incorporates anti inflammatory or acne-preventing components (e.G., niacinamide, salicylic acid, or tea tree oil).

Avoid heavy lotions or products with pore-clogging substances, at the side of petrolatum or mineral oil.

Apply a moisturizer times every day, following cleaning and every other pores and skin care treatments, to preserve healthful and hydrated pores and pores and skin. Remember that locating the right moisturizer in your pores and pores and skin can also additionally require some trial and errors, as genuinely each person's skin is specific. Don't be afraid to test with particular products until you find out one which works nicely in your pores and skin's dreams.

Sun Protection

Sun safety is a important component of any pores and pores and skin care ordinary, which encompass for people with pimples-willing pores and skin. While it can now not seem immediately associated with pimples, incorporating sun protection can assist prevent similarly harm and infection, sell pores and pores and skin recuperation, and reduce the risk of prolonged-time period pores and pores and skin troubles. In this segment, we will speak the significance of solar protection for acne-inclined pores and pores and skin and provide guidelines for choosing and making use of sunscreen.

1. Preventing hyperpigmentation and scarring: Acne can depart in the back of darkish spots and scars that take time to vanish. Sun exposure can worsen hyperpigmentation and make scars more important, because the solar's UV rays stimulate melanin production. Using giant-spectrum sunscreen can assist protect your pores and pores and skin and decrease the appearance of zits marks and scars.

2. Reducing irritation and infection: UV rays can motive contamination and infection, that can exacerbate gift zits and prevent the healing system. Protecting your skin from the sun permits to lessen

infection, permitting your pores and pores and pores and skin to heal more correctly.

3. Protecting towards premature developing older: Sun damage is a outstanding motive of untimely getting old, which embody wrinkles, great lines, and lack of elasticity. Using sunscreen frequently can help prevent those symptoms and signs and symptoms of growing vintage, ensuring that your pores and pores and skin remains wholesome and younger for longer.

four. Lowering pores and pores and skin most cancers threat: Regular use of sunscreen is vital for decreasing the danger of pores and pores and skin most cancers, including most cancers, the deadliest shape of pores and skin cancer. Acne-inclined skin is surely as susceptible to pores and pores and skin maximum cancers as each other pores and skin kind, so it is important to prioritize solar protection.

When selecting a sunscreen for acne-inclined pores and pores and skin, undergo in thoughts the following tips:

Opt for a wide-spectrum sunscreen with an SPF of 30 or better to guard in competition to each UVA and UVB rays.

Choose a light-weight, oil-loose, and non-comedogenic system that won't clog pores or exacerbate acne.

Look for sunscreens in particular designed for the face, as the ones are frequently extra appropriate for pimples-prone pores and skin.

Consider mineral or bodily sunscreens with zinc oxide or titanium dioxide, as they'll be an awful lot much less traumatic and pore-clogging than chemical sunscreens for some human beings.

In addition to the use of sunscreen, it is crucial to exercising special sun safety measures, including:

Reapplying sunscreen each hours or after swimming or sweating, even on cloudy days.

Wearing significant-brimmed hats, sun shades, and defensive clothing to shield your pores and pores and skin from the sun.

Seeking shade in some unspecified time in the future of top solar hours (10 a.M. To 4 p.M.) to decrease direct solar exposure

By incorporating sun safety into your every day skin care everyday, you will be taking an essential step closer to preserving healthy, easy pores and skin and reducing the hazard of lengthy-term pores and pores and skin damage.

Spot Treatments

Spot treatments are centered, concentrated products designed to deal with man or woman acne or zits lesions as they arise. They may be an crucial tool in your pimples-stopping arsenal, assisting to reduce the severity of breakouts, shorten their length, and prevent scarring. Spot treatments normally incorporate sturdy pimples-stopping substances that paintings to reduce irritation, kill zits-inflicting micro organism, and promote recovery. In this section, we are capable to talk some well-known spot treatment substances and a way to use them correctly.

1. Salicylic Acid: Salicylic acid is a beta-hydroxy acid (BHA) that might penetrate deep into the pores to dissolve extra oil, useless skin cells, and particles. It additionally has anti-inflammatory homes, making it an remarkable spot treatment preference for every inflammatory and non-inflammatory pimples.

2. Benzoyl Peroxide: Benzoyl peroxide is an antimicrobial agent that kills acne-causing bacteria (P. Acnes) with the beneficial resource of introducing oxygen into the pores. It can also assist to dry out acne and decrease infection, making it a famous preference for spot treatments.

three. Tea Tree Oil: Tea tree oil is a natural, plant-derived issue with antimicrobial and anti inflammatory homes. It can assist to lessen redness and contamination associated with acne, making it a gentler opportunity to benzoyl peroxide for a few people.

four. Sulfur: Sulfur is a herbal element with antibacterial and keratolytic residences, because of this it enables to interrupt down lifeless pores and pores and pores and skin cells and unclog pores. Sulfur spot remedies can assist to reduce the dimensions and severity of acne on the same time as also minimizing oil manufacturing.

five. Retinoids: Topical retinoids, such as adapalene or tretinoin, are derived from weight loss program A and can assist to unclog pores, reduce infection, and promote pores and skin cellular turnover. They may be used as spot treatments for zits-inclined skin, however their efficiency can also worsen some humans.

When the use of spot treatments, follow those guidelines for the wonderful results:

Apply the spot remedy immediately to the affected location after cleaning and in advance than moisturizing. Be superb to examine the product's specific commands for software program frequency and quantity.

Be affected individual and consistent. Some spot remedies may take some days to show consequences. Overusing the product or the use of an excessive amount of can aggravate and get worse acne.

Chapter 3: Natural Remedies for Acne

For the ones searching out alternative acne remedies or searching for to complement their present skin care ordinary, herbal remedies can provide a greater moderate, holistic method to dealing with acne. These treatments frequently harness the energy of plant-primarily based substances and herbal compounds to deal with infection, kill bacteria, and promote pores and pores and skin recovery. In this phase, we will find out a few famous natural remedies for pimples and their functionality benefits.

Tree Tea Oil:

Tea tree oil, moreover known as melaleuca oil, is an essential oil extracted from the leaves of the Melaleuca alternifolia plant, neighborhood to Australia. It has been used for masses of years as a herbal remedy for numerous pores and skin conditions, at the side of acne, due to its first rate antimicrobial, antifungal, and anti-inflammatory houses. The lively compounds in tea tree oil, which encompass terpinen-4-ol, are responsible for their efficacy in treating pimples and one of a kind pores and skin troubles.

Benefits of Tea Tree Oil for Acne:

1. Antimicrobial houses: Tea tree oil is effective in competition to many bacteria and fungi, which consist of Propionibacterium acnes, the micro organism accountable for causing pimples. By targeted on and getting rid of the ones micro organism, tea tree oil can help lessen the severity and frequency of breakouts.

2. Anti-inflammatory results: Acne is often placed by using using using redness and contamination, which can be painful and make a contribution to scarring. Tea tree oil has been established to lessen inflammation, helping to calm and soothe pimples-inclined pores and pores and pores and skin.

3. Unclogging pores: Tea tree oil can help to unclog pores by way of using manner of dissolving the oil, dirt, and useless pores and pores and skin cells which can acquire and reason breakouts. This makes it an powerful addition to zits-preventing pores and skin care bodily activities, supporting to save you new zits from forming.

4. Reducing pimples scars: Tea tree oil can also help to enhance the appearance of pimples scars through promoting pores and pores and pores and skin healing and lowering infection.

How to Use Tea Tree Oil for Acne:

When the usage of tea tree oil for pimples, it's crucial to dilute the critical oil in advance than making use of it to the pores and skin, as undiluted tea tree oil can motive contamination, dryness, or maybe burns.

1. Dilute tea tree oil with a service oil, inclusive of jojoba oil, sweet almond oil, or

grapeseed oil. A cutting-edge guideline is to combine 2-3 drops of tea tree oil with a teaspoon of carrier oil.

2. Apply the diluted tea tree oil right away to the affected region the usage of a cotton swab or clean fingertips. Avoid the usage of it to the encircling healthful skin, as this may motive useless infection.

3. Use tea tree oil a couple of instances every day, as needed, however show screen your pores and skin for symptoms and symptoms of irritation, together with redness, itching, or dryness. If you enjoy any unfavourable reactions, discontinue use or strive diluting the tea tree oil further.

four. Tea tree oil also can be decided in numerous skin care products, which include cleansers, toners, and see remedies, particularly formulated for zits-inclined skin.

Please phrase that even as tea tree oil can be an effective herbal remedy for zits, person outcomes can also range. If your acne is excessive or persistent, are searching for recommendation from a dermatologist for a custom designed treatment plan. Additionally, some humans can be allergic to tea tree oil, so it's far encouraged to carry out a patch take a look at earlier than applying it to your face.

Green Tea:

Green tea, derived from the leaves of the Camellia sinensis plant, has been fed on for hundreds of years for its numerous health advantages. Rich in antioxidants, in particular epigallocatechin gallate (EGCG), inexperienced tea has received popularity as a natural remedy for diverse pores and skin situations, which encompass pimples. Its anti inflammatory, antimicrobial, and antioxidant houses make it an powerful alternative for promoting wholesome, clean pores and pores and pores and skin.

Benefits of Green Tea for Acne:

1. Anti-inflammatory results: Green tea includes polyphenols, collectively with EGCG, that have powerful anti-inflammatory homes. These compounds can assist to lessen redness, contamination, and swelling associated with zits, presenting a relaxing impact at the pores and pores and pores and skin.

2. Antimicrobial residences: Green tea has been verified to exhibit antimicrobial interest in the route of Propionibacterium acnes, the micro organism accountable for causing pimples. By inhibiting the growth of acne-inflicting micro organism, inexperienced tea can assist to prevent and reduce breakouts.

3. Antioxidant protection: The antioxidants in green tea can assist to neutralize unfastened radicals, which might be molecules that could motive oxidative stress and harm to the pores and skin. By protective the skin from oxidative strain, green tea can help to prevent premature

developing antique and promote a clearer complexion.

4. Sebum regulation: Some research advocate that inexperienced tea can help to regulate sebum manufacturing, decreasing extra oil that could make contributions to clogged pores and acne formation.

How to Use Green Tea for Acne:

1. Green tea toner: Brew a cup of inexperienced tea and allow it cool. Soak a cotton ball or pad in the tea and lightly use it on your face as a toner after cleansing. Allow it to air dry, and then examine collectively together with your regular moisturizer. This can be completed a few times each day.

2. Green tea face masks: Mix 1-2 tablespoons of cooled, brewed green tea with identical factors uncooked honey to create a paste. Apply the aggregate to your face, heading off the attention area, and permit it take a seat for 10-15 minutes.

Rinse off with heat water and pat your face dry. Repeat 1-2 instances in step with week.

3. Green tea extract: Green tea extract can be determined in various skincare products, which encompass cleansers, moisturizers, and serums, specially formulated for acne-susceptible pores and pores and skin. Incorporate those products into your pores and skin care routine to harness the blessings of green tea.

four. Oral dietary supplements: Green tea dietary supplements, normally within the shape of pills or tablets, can be taken to promote normal health and pores and skin blessings. However, are looking for for advice from a healthcare professional earlier than which include any new nutritional dietary dietary supplements to your weight loss program.

Honey and Cinnamon

Honey and cinnamon are herbal substances that have been used for hundreds of years in conventional remedy for their fitness benefits. Both materials very own antimicrobial, anti-inflammatory, and antioxidant homes, making them a effective combination for treating zits-prone pores and pores and skin. (Test batch a small quantity in advance than the usage of!)

Benefits of Honey and Cinnamon for Acne:

1. Honey:

Antibacterial residences: Honey, mainly uncooked or Manuka honey, contains hydrogen peroxide and awesome compounds that exhibit antibacterial hobby closer to numerous micro organism, which incorporates Propionibacterium acnes.

Anti-inflammatory effects: Honey can help to assuage and decrease contamination associated with pimples, supplying remedy and selling the recuperation tool.

Antioxidant protection: Honey is wealthy in antioxidants, which could help to shield the pores and pores and skin from oxidative strain and sell a more healthy, clearer complexion.

Moisturizing and wound restoration: Honey is a herbal humectant, which means it can assist to preserve moisture within the pores and skin. It also has wound healing houses, that can help to decrease scarring and sell skin restore.

2. Cinnamon:

Antimicrobial houses: Cinnamon includes diverse lively compounds, such as cinnamaldehyde, that can help to inhibit the increase of pimples-inflicting bacteria and decrease the chance of breakouts.

Anti-inflammatory consequences: Cinnamon has been hooked up to showcase anti-inflammatory residences, assisting to reduce redness and swelling related to zits.

Antioxidant safety: Cinnamon is also wealthy in antioxidants, that could assist to shield the pores and pores and skin from oxidative stress and contribute to a clearer complexion.

How to Use Honey and Cinnamon for Acne:

1. Honey and cinnamon face mask: Mix one tablespoon of uncooked honey with half of a teaspoon of ground cinnamon to form a paste. Apply the mixture in your face, maintaining off the eye place, and permit it sit down down for 10-15 minutes. Rinse off with heat water and pat your face dry. Repeat 1-2 times consistent with week.

2. Honey and cinnamon spot treatment: Combine identical additives uncooked honey and ground cinnamon to create a thick paste. Apply the aggregate proper away to the affected vicinity using a cotton swab or easy fingertips. Leave it on for 15-20 minutes, or in a single day for extra severe zits, then rinse with heat water. Use as needed.

Aloe Vera

Aloe vera, a succulent plant species, has been used for masses of years for its numerous health and medicinal homes. The clean gel extracted from its leaves is rich in vitamins, minerals, enzymes, and amino acids, making it a popular choice for treating a big variety of skin situations, such as zits. Aloe vera's soothing, anti inflammatory, and antimicrobial homes make it an effective natural treatment for zits-willing pores and skin.

Benefits of Aloe Vera for Acne:

1. Anti-inflammatory results: Aloe vera consists of compounds collectively with glycoproteins and polysaccharides that exhibit anti inflammatory houses. These compounds assist to lessen redness, swelling, and infection associated with zits, supplying relief and selling recuperation.

2. Antimicrobial homes: Aloe vera has been tested to very very own antimicrobial interest in the course of severa bacteria,

together with Propionibacterium acnes, the primary bacteria liable for inflicting acne. By inhibiting the boom of zits-inflicting micro organism, aloe vera can help to save you and reduce breakouts.

3. Soothing and cooling consequences: Aloe vera is thought for its soothing and cooling outcomes on the pores and skin, which can offer relief for irritated or inflamed acne-susceptible pores and pores and skin.

4. Promotes pores and skin recovery: Aloe vera carries nutrients, enzymes, and minerals that can assist to stimulate pores and pores and skin cellular regeneration and sell the recuperation method. This may be in particular beneficial for decreasing the advent of acne scars and improving commonplace pores and pores and skin texture.

5. Moisturizing blessings: Aloe vera is a natural humectant, this means that that it

could assist to hold moisture inside the pores and pores and skin with out clogging pores or causing oiliness. This makes it a super moisturizer for zits-inclined pores and pores and pores and skin sorts.

How to Use Aloe Vera for Acne:

1. Pure aloe vera gel: Apply natural aloe vera gel without delay to the affected vicinity or use it as an all-over facial moisturizer. You should purchase aloe vera gel from fitness stores or extract it from the leaves of an aloe vera plant. Ensure that the product you choose out is freed from brought fragrances, shades, or different irritants.

2. Aloe vera-infused skincare merchandise: Many pores and skin care merchandise, along aspect cleansers, toners, and moisturizers, incorporate aloe vera as a key detail. Incorporate those products into your skin care habitual to

harness the blessings of aloe vera for pimples-inclined skin.

three. DIY aloe vera face mask: Combine 1-2 tablespoons of herbal aloe vera gel with 1 tablespoon of honey or some drops of tea tree oil. Apply the mixture in your face, keeping off the attention location, and allow it take a seat down down for 15-20 minutes. Rinse off with heat water and pat your face dry. Repeat 1-2 instances regular with week.

Apple Cider Vinegar

Apple cider vinegar (ACV) is a fermented liquid made from beaten apples, sugar, and yeast. It has been used for hundreds of years for severa fitness blessings, which incorporates pores and skin care. ACV includes acetic, citric, and malic acids, similarly to useful enzymes, vitamins, and minerals that make it a popular herbal remedy for pimples-willing pores and pores and skin.

Benefits of Apple Cider Vinegar for Acne:

1. Antimicrobial houses: Apple cider vinegar has been confirmed to possess antimicrobial interest toward some of micro organism and fungi, inclusive of Propionibacterium acnes, the bacteria liable for causing pimples. By inhibiting the growth of acne-inflicting micro organism, ACV can help to save you and decrease breakouts.

2. Balancing pores and skin pH: The natural acids found in apple cider vinegar can assist to stability the pores and pores and pores and skin's pH, which may additionally create an surroundings masses much much less favorable for pimples-causing micro organism to thrive. Balanced pores and pores and skin pH can also assist to regulate sebum production, lowering excess oil that would make contributions to clogged pores and acne formation.

3. Exfoliation: The herbal acids in ACV can lightly exfoliate the pores and pores and skin, casting off useless pores and pores and skin cells and debris that might clog pores

and cause breakouts. Regular exfoliation can help to sell a clearer, smoother complexion.

four. Reducing infection and redness: Apple cider vinegar has anti inflammatory homes that could help to assuage and decrease infection and redness associated with zits.

How to Use Apple Cider Vinegar for Acne:

1. ACV toner: Mix one part uncooked, unfiltered apple cider vinegar with elements water to create a diluted answer. Soak a cotton ball or pad in the solution and gently use it on your face as a toner after cleaning. Allow it to air dry, and then have a look at collectively along with your normal moisturizer. This can be carried out a few instances each day. If your pores and pores and skin is sensitive, remember diluting the ACV in addition or the use of it plenty less often.

2. ACV spot treatment: Mix equal additives uncooked, unfiltered apple cider vinegar with water. Apply the diluted answer proper now to the affected place using a cotton swab or smooth fingertips. Leave it on for 15-20 minutes, or in a single day for greater extreme pimples, after which rinse off with heat water. Use as needed.

three. ACV face mask: Combine 1 tablespoon of uncooked, unfiltered apple cider vinegar with 2 tablespoons of bentonite clay or inexperienced clay. Mix well to shape a smooth paste. Apply the aggregate in your face, retaining off the attention location, and allow it sit down down for 10-15 minutes. Rinse off with warmth water and pat your face dry. Repeat 1-2 times ordinary with week.

Chapter 4: The Importance of Lifestyle In Acne Prevention

A complete approach to zits prevention and treatment consists of no longer handiest a right pores and skin care ordinary and eating regimen but moreover a healthful manner of existence. Various life-style elements, inclusive of pressure, sleep, exercising, and hydration, play a important feature in pores and pores and pores and skin health and can make a contribution to the development and severity of acne. This section will speak the importance of those elements and offer some tips on a way to preserve a balanced life-style for clearer, more healthy pores and skin

Stress Management and Relaxation Techniques

Effectively coping with pressure is critical for common fitness and nicely-being, which include pores and pores and skin fitness. As formerly noted, stress can cause an increase in cortisol manufacturing, that might contribute to pimples breakouts. Incorporating relaxation strategies into your daily recurring will let you control strain and promote a extra healthful complexion. Here are some strain manipulate and relaxation techniques to go through in thoughts:

1. Deep Breathing Exercises: Practicing deep breathing bodily sports activities can assist activate your body's relaxation response, reduce stress degrees, and calm your thoughts. One well-known technique is diaphragmatic respiratory or belly respiratory. To workout this method, sit or lie down in a comfortable role, and place one hand on your chest and the opposite in your belly. Inhale slowly through your nose, allowing your stomach to upward push as you fill your lungs with air. Exhale slowly via your mouth or nostril, allowing your stomach to fall. Repeat this technique for numerous minutes, focusing in your breath.

2. Meditation: Meditation is a exercising that allows to calm the thoughts and

promote relaxation. There are many styles of meditation, which includes mindfulness meditation, guided meditation, and loving-kindness meditation. To begin, discover a quiet, cushty region in which you can sit or lie down. Focus in your breath or a particular issue of interest, and let your thoughts bypass with the useful resource of the use of with out judgment. Begin with quick periods of five-10 minutes and frequently growth the length as you turn out to be extra snug with the exercise.

3. Yoga: Yoga is a thoughts-frame exercise that mixes bodily postures, breathing wearing sports, and meditation to promote relaxation and strain discount. Regular yoga exercise can help enhance flexibility, electricity, and highbrow readability. Consider becoming a member of a neighborhood yoga splendor or following online yoga tutorials to get started out.

4. Progressive Muscle Relaxation (PMR): PMR is a manner that includes tensing and

enjoyable specific muscle groups in a systematic order. This practice can help to release tension from your body and promote relaxation. To exercise PMR, discover a quiet, comfortable area in which you may take a seat down or lie down. Starting collectively with your ft and strolling your way up to your face, disturbing each muscle institution for 5-10 seconds after which lighten up for 15-20 seconds. Focus on the sensation of tension and rest in every muscle institution.

5. Engage in Enjoyable Activities: Make time for interests and sports that convey you pleasure and rest. Whether it is painting, playing an tool, gardening, or spending time in nature, wearing out activities you experience can assist to lessen stress and sell a pleasing nation of thoughts.

6. Social Support: Connecting with supportive pals, family contributors, or a therapist will let you manipulate strain via offering an outlet to proportion your

emotions and communicate strategies to manage. Building sturdy social connections can contribute to normal emotional well-being and stress reduce fee.

Remember that strain control is a non-public journey, and special techniques paintings for particular people. Experiment with diverse rest techniques to discover those who paintings high-quality for you and make them a regular a part of your every day habitual. By efficiently coping with stress, you could useful resource your pores and skin's health and artwork towards zits prevention.

The Impact of Sleep

Adequate sleep is critical for common fitness, along with the health of your pores and skin. During sleep, your body undergoes numerous restorative techniques that make a contribution to keeping a wholesome complexion and stopping zits breakouts.

Here's a deeper take a look at the effect of sleep on pores and pores and skin fitness:

1.   Skin Repair and Regeneration: While you sleep, your body works to repair damaged pores and pores and skin cells, regenerate new cells, and replace older cells. This way lets in to maintain the overall health and appearance of your pores and skin. A loss of sleep can disrupt this natural restore technique, main to a dull, worn-out-searching complexion and probably contributing to the improvement of pimples.

2.   Reduced Inflammation: Sleep plays a critical position in regulating your frame's inflammatory response. During sleep, the producing of anti-inflammatory molecules will growth, helping to lessen irritation at some point of the body, including the pores and pores and pores and skin. Insufficient sleep can make contributions to stepped forward infection, which might also additionally exacerbate gift pimples and put

off the restoration way of present blemishes.

3. Hormone Regulation: Hormones play a terrific function inside the development and severity of pimples. Sleep permits to adjust the producing of severa hormones, in conjunction with cortisol, insulin, and growth hormone. A lack of sleep can cause hormonal imbalances, which may additionally additionally make contributions to improved sebum production, irritation, and acne improvement.

four. Enhanced Immune Function: Sleep is essential for preserving a wholesome immune gadget, which lets in to protect your pores and pores and pores and skin from zits-causing bacteria and specific pathogens. Insufficient sleep can weaken your immune device, making it more tough in your frame to combat off infections, together with people who make a contribution to pimples.

5. Stress Reduction: Adequate sleep can assist to lessen strain stages, which, as previously noted, can make contributions to the improvement of pimples. By making sure proper sleep, you can better manage strain and reduce its effect for your skin.

To optimize sleep for better pores and skin fitness, don't forget the subsequent suggestions:

Establish a constant sleep time desk via going to mattress and waking up on the equal time each day, even on weekends.

Create a relaxing bedtime normal to signal your body that it is time to wind down. This may encompass taking a warmness tub, analyzing a e-book, or schooling relaxation strategies.

Make your sleep environment conducive to relaxation with the useful resource of ensuring it's miles darkish, quiet, and at a snug temperature.

Limit publicity to digital gadgets as a minimum one hour earlier than bedtime, because of the truth the blue mild emitted can interfere at the aspect of your herbal sleep cycle.

Consider enforcing strain manage strategies, as stress can negatively effect the quality of your sleep.

By prioritizing sleep and maintaining a consistent sleep time desk, you may useful resource your pores and skin's fitness and work inside the path of acne prevention.

Exercise and Skin Health

Regular workout gives severa health blessings, which includes advanced pores and pores and skin health. Physical interest can make contributions to a greater healthful, greater balanced complexion with the aid of manner of manner of promoting blood flow into, decreasing stress, and regulating hormone stages. Here's a higher study the impact of workout on skin fitness:

1. Increased Blood Circulation: Exercise will growth blood go together with the go with the flow at some degree within the body, collectively with the pores and skin. Enhanced blood waft gives oxygen and crucial nutrients to pores and skin cells, selling trendy pores and pores and skin health and supporting to keep a greater youthful, radiant appearance. Improved blood go with the drift also aids in the elimination of pollutants and waste products from pores and skin cells, supporting the natural detoxification gadget.

2. Reduced Stress: Engaging in regular bodily interest is a tested manner to reduce stress levels. As formerly stated, strain can contribute to the development of acne through increasing cortisol production and causing hormonal imbalances. By incorporating exercising into your normal, you may control stress greater efficiently and decrease its impact to your skin.

3. Hormone Regulation: Exercise can assist alter hormone stages, together with insulin and cortisol, which play a feature in acne improvement. Regular physical interest can beautify insulin sensitivity, supporting to hold robust blood sugar ranges and reduce contamination. Additionally, exercising can assist lower cortisol tiers, which might also additionally reduce sebum manufacturing and reduce the opportunity of acne breakouts.

4. Improved Immune Function: Regular workout can enhance your immune tool, improving your frame's capability to combat off infections and protect your pores and skin from pimples-causing bacteria. A robust immune machine helps general pores and pores and skin health and lets in to maintain a easy complexion.

five. Sweating and Detoxification: Sweating during workout can assist flush out impurities and pollution out of your pores and skin, clearing your pores and decreasing the risk of clogged pores and pimples formation. However, it's far important to cleanse your face after workout to get rid of sweat and micro organism that might make contributions to breakouts.

To incorporate exercising into your everyday for better pores and skin health, keep in mind the following hints:

Aim for as a minimum one hundred and fifty mins of slight-depth aerobic hobby or 75 mins of lively-depth cardio interest consistent with week, as encouraged with the useful resource of the American Heart Association.

Choose activities which you enjoy and might effortlessly suit into some time desk. This may additionally encompass taking walks, jogging, swimming, biking, dancing, or participating in employer fitness instructions.

Incorporate strength training carrying occasions as a minimum days steady with week to enhance muscle energy and tone, that could beautify your normal look.

Listen for your frame and modify your exercise regular as desired. Over-workout can bring about physical stress and probable exacerbate pores and pores and skin issues. Find a stability that works for you and promotes traditional properly-being.

By making workout a everyday part of your way of life, you may guide your pores and skin's health and artwork within the route of pimples prevention. Remember that consistency is fundamental, and it is able to take time to look the whole advantages of exercise in your pores and pores and skin.

Hydration and its Effect on Acne

Proper hydration are crucial for widespread health, which include the health of your pores and pores and skin. While staying hydrated might not straight away prevent pimples, it performs a vital feature in maintaining a healthful, balanced complexion. Here's a better check the consequences of hydration on zits and pores and pores and skin fitness:

1. Skin Elasticity and Radiance: Drinking sufficient water lets in maintain your pores and pores and skin's elasticity, stopping dryness and flakiness. Well-hydrated pores and pores and skin appears plumper and further radiant, as water lets in to fill the areas between pores and skin cells and keep a easy ground.

2. Detoxification: Proper hydration aids within the natural detoxification approach via supporting kidney function and promoting the removal of waste merchandise and pollution from the frame. By flushing out impurities, you can assist preserve easy, healthful pores and skin and potentially reduce the danger of pimples formation.

3. Skin Barrier Function: Adequate hydration is crucial for keeping a healthful pores and skin barrier. A well-functioning pores and skin barrier allows to lock in moisture and save you water loss, defensive the pores and skin from outside irritants and pathogens, which encompass pimples-inflicting micro organism.

4. Reduced Inflammation: Staying hydrated can help reduce inflammation inside the frame, that is mainly beneficial for humans with acne-willing pores and pores and skin. Chronic inflammation can exacerbate pimples and delay the healing process. Drinking sufficient water can assist to balance your frame's inflammatory reaction and assist everyday pores and pores and pores and skin health.

5. Sebum Production Regulation: Although the direct relationship among hydration and sebum production is not however actually understood, staying hydrated may also make contributions to a

more balanced sebum manufacturing. When the pores and skin is dehydrated, it could produce extra oil to atone for the lack of moisture, fundamental to clogged pores and acne.

To stay nicely hydrated and help healthful pores and skin, take into account the following recommendations:

Aim to drink at the least 8-10 cups (sixty 4-eighty oz.) of water steady with day, or more in case you're bodily active or stay in a warm climate. Individual water consumption necessities may additionally additionally variety based on elements which includes age, sex, and everyday fitness.

Incorporate water-rich culmination and vegetables into your eating regimen. Some examples consist of cucumbers, watermelons, strawberries, oranges, and grapefruit. These food can assist to increase your each day water intake and provide vital nutrients and minerals for pores and pores and skin fitness.

Limit your consumption of diuretics, consisting of caffeine and alcohol, that can make contributions to dehydration. If you do devour those beverages, make sure to drink extra water to atone for the fluid loss.

Monitor your urine color as a stylish gauge of your hydration popularity. Ideally, your urine have to be a light, straw-like coloration. Darker urine can advocate dehydration and the want to boom your water intake.

By specializing in proper hydration, you could useful resource your pores and pores and skin's health and contribute to a extra balanced, acne-resistant complexion. Remember that accomplishing and retaining clean pores and pores and skin is a holistic approach that calls for ordinary attempt and interest to numerous manner of lifestyles factors.

Chapter 5: Medical Treatments for Acne

While manner of life modifications and herbal remedies may be effective in coping with zits for some people, others also can require clinical intervention to deal with their situation. A dermatologist can assist decide the maximum suitable route of motion primarily based at the severity and shape of pimples. In this section, we're capable of discover common medical remedies for zits.

Over-the-Counter Treatments

Over-the-counter (OTC) remedies are substantially to be had and may be an powerful first-line technique for humans with moderate to moderate pimples. These remedies frequently contain energetic components that artwork to unclog pores, lessen inflammation, and combat acne-causing bacteria. Here's a better take a look at some not unusual OTC zits treatments and their functions:

1. Benzoyl Peroxide: Benzoyl peroxide is a famous OTC acne remedy to be had in diverse concentrations (usually 2.Five% to ten%). It works with the aid of killing pimples-causing bacteria, reducing contamination, and unclogging pores. Benzoyl peroxide may be placed in cleansers, lotions, gels, and spot remedies. It's vital initially a lower attention to limit pores and skin infection and regularly growth as wanted. Keep in mind that benzoyl peroxide may additionally bleach fabric, so be cautious at the equal time as using it near garb, towels, or bedding.

2. Salicylic Acid: Salicylic acid is a beta-hydroxy acid (BHA) that enables to unclog pores via the use of breaking down vain pores and skin cells and extra oil. It additionally has anti inflammatory houses, making it powerful in treating acne-willing pores and pores and skin. Salicylic acid can be determined in numerous paperwork, in conjunction with cleansers, toners, gels, and

notice treatments, commonly at concentrations starting from zero.Five% to two%. It's vital to conform with the product's hints and be affected man or woman, as it is able to take several weeks to appearance superb enhancements.

3. Alpha-Hydroxy Acids (AHAs): Alpha-hydroxy acids, which incorporates glycolic acid and lactic acid, are usually found in OTC acne remedies. These acids art work thru exfoliating the skin, removing dead pores and pores and skin cells, and selling mobile turnover. This method allows to unclog pores, reduce the advent of zits scars, and enhance pores and skin texture. AHAs can be determined in cleansers, toners, lotions, and serums. As with other OTC remedies, it's far important to have a look at the product's recommendations and be affected person, as it is able to take time to appearance enhancements.

four. Sulfur: Sulfur is every other detail that may be located in some OTC pimples treatments. It works with the useful resource of manner of drying out more oil, unclogging pores, and lowering infection. Sulfur is often blended with distinct acne-preventing components, in conjunction with benzoyl peroxide or salicylic acid, to beautify its effectiveness. While sulfur may be effective for a few human beings, it may cause pores and pores and skin contamination or an ugly fragrance for others.

five. Niacinamide: Niacinamide, a shape of vitamins B3, has acquired reputation as an OTC acne remedy because of its anti-inflammatory houses and capacity to alter sebum production. It can help to reduce redness, infection, and the arrival of pimples lesions. Niacinamide can be determined in numerous pores and pores and skin care products, along side serums, lotions, and toners.

When the use of OTC acne remedies, it's miles important to observe the product's directions and be affected person, as it can take several weeks to peer enormous improvements. Additionally, it's miles crucial to patch-test any new product on a small vicinity of pores and pores and skin earlier than the usage of it on your entire face to make certain you do now not have an poor reaction. If you find out that OTC treatments are not supplying the popular effects, or if your acne worsens, it is essential to visit a dermatologist to speak approximately opportunity treatment alternatives.

Prescription Medications

When over the counter remedies fail to offer first rate consequences or if an individual has more intense or continual acne, a dermatologist may also moreover moreover prescribe more potent drug remedies. Prescription medicinal drugs for zits can be more potent and centered, assisting to address the underlying causes of the situation. Here's a top degree view of some common prescription medicinal pills for zits:

1. Oral Antibiotics: Oral antibiotics, such as tetracycline, doxycycline, minocycline, and erythromycin, may be prescribed to deal with mild to excessive acne, specifically even as inflammation and infection are gift. These medications art work through lowering infection and killing zits-inflicting micro organism. Oral antibiotics are commonly prescribed for a restrained length (usually some months) to avoid antibiotic resistance. It's crucial to comply at the side of your healthcare organisation's commands while the use of antibiotics and to finish the entire path, even in case your zits clears up in advance than the drugs is finished.

2. Topical Antibiotics: Topical antibiotics, like clindamycin and erythromycin, are applied proper now to the pores and pores and skin to intention zits-inflicting bacteria and reduce

inflammation. These medicinal pills are regularly prescribed in combination with unique acne treatments, together with benzoyl peroxide or a topical retinoid, to decorate their effectiveness and decrease the danger of antibiotic resistance. As with oral antibiotics, it's important to have a study your healthcare organisation's commands while using topical antibiotics.

3. Oral Retinoids: Oral retinoids, which incorporates isotretinoin (normally acknowledged via manner of its former emblem name, Accutane), are normally reserved for the most excessive instances of acne that have no longer responded to other treatments. Isotretinoin works with the useful resource of reducing oil manufacturing, contamination, and clogged pores. Due to its efficiency and capacity issue outcomes, isotretinoin is usually prescribed for a restrained length (normally 4-6 months) below near supervision with the useful useful resource of a

dermatologist. Patients ought to examine strict hints and take part in a chance management software (iPledge in the United States) because of the capacity for immoderate transport defects if taken at some stage in being pregnant.

4. Topical Retinoids: Topical retinoids, which incorporates tretinoin, adapalene, and tazarotene, are prescription-power medicinal drugs derived from vitamins A. These remedies assist to unclog pores, reduce infection, and promote cell turnover, number one to clearer pores and pores and skin. It's essential to comply together with your dermatologist's commands at the same time as using topical retinoids, as they might purpose pores and skin irritation, dryness, and improved solar sensitivity. Start with a lower interest and often increase as desired, and always follow sunscreen in some unspecified time in the future of the day to protect your pores and skin from sun harm.

5. Hormonal Therapy: For women experiencing hormonal acne, hormonal remedy, together with oral contraceptives or anti-androgen medicinal pills (e.G., spironolactone), may be effective in treating pimples. These medicines assist to regulate hormone ranges, lowering sebum manufacturing and zits breakouts. Your healthcare organization will determine if hormonal treatment is appropriate for you primarily based definitely in your medical facts, specific dreams, and ability aspect effects.

6. Azelaic Acid: Azelaic acid is a prescription medicine that works by way of reducing infection, killing pimples-causing bacteria, and unclogging pores. It's mainly useful for humans with sensitive pores and skin, as it has a tendency to be gentler than particular zits treatments. Azelaic acid is available as a cream or gel and must be achieved as directed through your healthcare enterprise.

When using prescription drugs for acne, it's critical to comply with your healthcare organization's instructions and attend everyday have a observe-up appointments to screen your progress and modify your remedy plan as desired. It's important to be affected character, as it could take numerous weeks or months to see superb upgrades to your pores and pores and pores and skin's look. Always talk any issues or facet consequences with

Topical Retinoids

Topical retinoids are a class of prescription-strength drugs derived from nutrients A this is typically used to address pimples. They art work via manner of unclogging pores, lowering infection, and promoting mobile turnover, which allows to clean present zits and save you new breakouts. Topical retinoids have additionally been shown to beautify pores and skin texture and reduce the arrival of zits scars. Some of the most generally prescribed topical retinoids include:

1. Tretinoin: Tretinoin (additionally referred to as Retin-A or Renova) is one of the most notably prescribed topical retinoids for treating pimples. It is to be had in severa concentrations and formulations, together with lotions, gels, and creams. Tretinoin works through promoting the losing of dull pores and pores and skin cells, stimulating collagen production, and lowering infection.

2. Adapalene: Adapalene (logo call Differin) is a greater moderen-technology topical retinoid this is powerful in treating slight to mild acne. It is available each over-the-counter (at a decrease hobby) and by using manner of manner of prescription. Adapalene is thought for being gentler on the pores and pores and skin than some different retinoids, making it a amazing preference for individuals with sensitive pores and pores and skin.

3. Tazarotene: Tazarotene (brand names Tazorac, Fabior) is any other topical retinoid that is effective in treating pimples. It is to be had as a cream or gel in various concentrations. Tazarotene is generally prescribed for slight to excessive pimples and has been tested to be especially effective in treating inflammatory acne lesions.

When the usage of topical retinoids, it's miles vital to conform together with your dermatologist's instructions, as they are capable of motive pores and skin contamination, dryness, and prolonged solar sensitivity. Here are a few recommendations for using topical retinoids efficiently and appropriately:

Start with a lower recognition and step by step boom as desired. Your dermatologist may additionally moreover moreover prescribe a decrease attention to start with and alter it over the years based absolutely in your pores and skin's tolerance and reaction to the drugs.

Apply a small amount of the product to easy, dry skin. Using an excessive amount of retinoid can boom the threat of infection without offering additional advantages.

Use topical retinoids at night time time time, as they will degrade and lose effectiveness at the same time as exposed to sunlight hours.

Apply a sizable-spectrum sunscreen with an SPF of 30 or higher each day, as topical retinoids could make your pores and skin more touchy to the sun.

Be affected man or woman, as it may take numerous weeks or possibly months to look essential enhancements for your pores and skin's appearance. It isn't unusual for acne to appear worse earlier than it gets higher, due to the fact the retinoids supply underlying zits to the floor.

Be aware about functionality aspect consequences, which include redness, peeling, dryness, or itching. If those facet results are extreme or chronic, contact your dermatologist for advice on a way to manipulate them or whether or not to alter your treatment plan.

By using topical retinoids as directed and working towards accurate skincare behavior, many human beings with acne can revel in large upgrades in their pores and skin's look and usual fitness.

Antibiotics

Antibiotics are medicinal drugs used to deal with bacterial infections, and additionally they may be effective in treating acne. They paintings through using decreasing infection and centered on the pimples-inflicting micro organism, Propionibacterium acnes (P. Acnes). Antibiotics can be prescribed in oral or topical shape, depending on the severity of the pimples and the person's precise wishes. Here's a pinnacle level view of some commonplace antibiotics used for zits treatment:

Oral Antibiotics:

1. Tetracycline: Tetracycline is an oral antibiotic often prescribed for pimples because of its anti-inflammatory and antibacterial houses. It is normally used for slight to immoderate acne and is generally taken for several weeks to three months. Possible thing outcomes encompass gastrointestinal disenchanted, sensitivity to daylight, and, in uncommon times, enamel discoloration in children.

2. Doxycycline: Doxycycline is a by-product of tetracycline and is a few unique oral antibiotic usually prescribed for pimples. It is effective in treating inflammatory pimples and is often applied in mixture with different acne remedies. Side consequences can encompass gastrointestinal disenchanted, sun

sensitivity, and, in uncommon times, an advanced danger of a immoderate pores and pores and skin reaction known as drug-delivered approximately allergy syndrome.

3. Minocycline: Minocycline is a few different derivative of tetracycline and is regularly prescribed for moderate to severe pimples. It has a slightly awesome spectrum of hobby in assessment to doxycycline, making it effective towards a few resistant traces of P. Acnes. Potential aspect outcomes consist of gastrointestinal disenchanted, dizziness, and, in uncommon times, a bluish discoloration of the pores and pores and skin or teeth.

4. Erythromycin: Erythromycin is a macrolide antibiotic that can be prescribed for acne even as tetracyclines aren't suitable, together with in some unspecified time in the future of being pregnant or for humans with a tetracycline hypersensitive reaction. Erythromycin is typically well-tolerated, however component results can

also include gastrointestinal disenchanted and the development of antibiotic resistance.

Topical Antibiotics:

1. Clindamycin: Clindamycin is a topical antibiotic this is powerful in treating acne by means of the use of decreasing inflammation and focused on P. Acnes micro organism. It is regularly prescribed in mixture with benzoyl peroxide or a topical retinoid to decorate its effectiveness and reduce the risk of antibiotic resistance. Side consequences may moreover encompass dryness, redness, and infection at the software net web site.

2. Erythromycin: Erythromycin is also available as a topical antibiotic for zits remedy. Similar to clindamycin, it works thru reducing infection and concentrated on P. Acnes bacteria. It is regularly blended with benzoyl peroxide or notable zits remedies to increase efficacy and decrease

antibiotic resistance. Side consequences can also include redness, dryness, and infection at the software internet web web page.

When the use of antibiotics for pimples, it is crucial to conform along with your healthcare company's instructions and complete the entire path of treatment, even in case your acne clears up before the medicine is completed. This permits to prevent antibiotic resistance and ensures the handiest remedy possible. Additionally, it is critical to speak any problems or side consequences together with your healthcare organization, as they'll want to adjust your remedy plan or prescribe an possibility medicinal drug. Remember that antibiotics are excellent one a part of a complete pimples treatment plan, which may additionally furthermore encompass topical treatments, life-style changes, and remarkable medicinal capsules.

Hormonal Therapy

Hormonal remedy may be an effective remedy for women experiencing hormonal zits, this is often characterized with the useful resource of breakouts taking place throughout the menstrual cycle, along the jawline, and at the chin. Hormonal treatment works with the useful resource of regulating hormone levels, specially androgens, which can be male hormones observed in every women and men that could stimulate sebum production and make a contribution to zits improvement. Here's a pinnacle stage view of a few not unusual hormonal treatments used for zits treatment:

1. Oral Contraceptives: Oral contraceptives, or starting manipulate drugs, can help adjust hormone ranges in girls and are regularly prescribed for the treatment of hormonal zits. The pills commonly incorporate a aggregate of estrogen and progestin, that might assist suppress the ovaries' manufacturing of

androgens. The U.S. Food and Drug Administration (FDA) has approved numerous oral contraceptives mainly for pimples treatment, which embody Ortho Tri-Cyclen, Estrostep, and Yaz. It's essential to searching for advice out of your healthcare company to decide if oral contraceptives are a suitable remedy desire in your acne and talk functionality facet consequences and risks. Some commonplace thing effects of oral contraceptives encompass weight gain, temper swings, and, in unusual times, an increased threat of blood clots.

2. Anti-Androgen Medications: Anti-androgen tablets, which consist of spironolactone, artwork thru manner of blockading the effects of androgens on the sebaceous glands, reducing sebum production, and in the end decreasing zits breakouts. Spironolactone is commonly prescribed off-label for hormonal zits treatment, specially for ladies who enjoy

acne flares round their menstrual cycle or have polycystic ovary syndrome (PCOS). As with oral contraceptives, it's crucial to seek advice from your healthcare company to determine if anti-androgen medicinal capsules are appropriate in your specific desires and communicate capability element outcomes and dangers. Some commonplace side effects of spironolactone encompass dizziness, expanded urination, and, in uncommon cases, an extended potassium degree inside the blood.

When the use of hormonal treatment for acne, it's far important to comply at the side of your healthcare issuer's instructions and attend regular take a look at-up appointments to reveal your improvement and modify your remedy plan as wanted. It's essential to be patient, as it could take severa months to look major enhancements to your pores and skin's appearance. Additionally, constantly communicate any troubles or facet consequences together with your healthcare business enterprise, as they'll want to alter your remedy plan or prescribe an opportunity treatment. Hormonal treatment can be an vital part of a whole zits remedy plan, which may consist of topical treatments, lifestyle adjustments, and one-of-a-kind drugs.

Chemical Peels and Microdermabrasion

Chemical peels and microdermabrasion are non-invasive, expert pores and pores and skin treatments that can be powerful in handling zits and improving pores and skin texture. These treatments artwork via using getting rid of the outermost layers of the pores and skin to expose a smoother, more even complexion. While every remedies can be useful for pimples-inclined skin, they address fantastic concerns and use outstanding techniques.

Chemical Peels:

Chemical peels include making use of a chemical solution, commonly containing acids like glycolic, salicylic, or lactic acid, to the pores and skin's ground. The solution motives the pinnacle layers of the skin to peel off, revealing more energizing, greater healthy skin under. Chemical peels can help lessen zits breakouts, fade pimples scars, and decorate not unusual pores and skin texture. The intensity of a chemical peel can variety from light to deep, counting on the sort and cognizance of the acid used and the desired outcomes. Some blessings of chemical peels for zits-inclined pores and skin encompass:

Exfoliation of lifeless pores and skin cells, that may assist unclog pores and save you acne breakouts

Reducing contamination and redness related to acne

Stimulating collagen manufacturing, that could improve the appearance of pimples scars

Some capacity aspect effects of chemical peels encompass redness, peeling, and, in unusual instances, scarring or discoloration. It's important to are looking for recommendation from an authorized professional, which include a dermatologist or esthetician, for a chemical peel and to comply with their aftercare instructions to make certain right healing and maximum beneficial outcomes.

Microdermabrasion:

Microdermabrasion is a mechanical exfoliation technique that includes using a tool to softly dispose of the pinnacle layer of pores and skin, promoting cell turnover and revealing a smoother, greater even complexion. This remedy can help unclog pores, lessen the advent of zits scars, and improve regular pores and skin texture. Microdermabrasion is commonly suitable for all pores and pores and skin kinds, and the remedy may be customized to cope with character pores and skin worries. Some advantages of microdermabrasion for pimples-prone pores and skin consist of:

Gentle exfoliation that facilitates unclog pores and prevent breakouts

Reducing the appearance of pimples scars with the resource of selling collagen production

Improving average pores and skin texture and tone

Potential side effects of microdermabrasion are commonly moderate and may encompass short redness, dryness, or sensitivity. As with chemical peels, it is crucial to are in search of for advice from a certified expert for a microdermabrasion treatment and have a examine their aftercare instructions for the first-rate outcomes.

Both chemical peels and microdermabrasion can be effective treatments for pimples-susceptible skin whilst carried out via a certified professional and combined with a complete pimples treatment plan, collectively with proper skincare, way of existence adjustments, and, if vital, greater scientific remedies. It's essential to attempting to find recommendation from a dermatologist or skincare professional to determine which treatment is most suitable on your specific skin concerns and desires.

Chapter 6: Preventing Acne Scars and Treating Existing Scars

Acne scars might also moreover have a full-size effect on an individual's self-self notion and widely wide-spread nicely-being. Therefore, it's far critical to take steps to prevent zits scars and deal with current scars successfully. This phase will speak pointers for preventing pimples scars, topical treatments for scarring, and expert treatments for acne scars.

Tips for Preventing Acne Scars:

Preventing zits scars starts offevolved offevolved with proper pimples manipulate and pores and skin care habits. By taking steps to lessen breakouts and infection, you may decrease the risk of scarring. Here are some improved tips for preventing pimples scars:

1. Do now not pick out or squeeze pimples: Resisting the urge to pick out out or squeeze pimples lesions is vital. Picking at

your pores and pores and skin can motive inflammation, contamination, and capability skin damage, foremost to scars. Instead, use spot treatments containing salicylic acid or benzoyl peroxide to assist accelerate the healing approach without causing in addition damage.

2. Treat acne early: Addressing acne as fast as it seems can help reduce the severity and duration of breakouts, which in turn minimizes the chance of scarring. Consult a dermatologist or skin care expert to increase a entire remedy plan tailored on your specific wishes, and observe their suggestions continuously.

3. Maintain a normal pores and skin care ordinary: A constant skin care habitual can assist save you breakouts and decrease the threat of scarring. Focus on mild cleaning, exfoliating, and moisturizing with merchandise designed on your pores and pores and skin type. Avoid harsh, abrasive products that can reason pores and pores

and skin infection and get worse zits. Additionally, make certain which you're doing away with make-up and excess oil out of your pores and skin every night time earlier than bed.

four. Use non-comedogenic products: Non-comedogenic products are designed now not to clog pores, which could help save you zits breakouts and decrease the threat of scarring. Look for pores and skin care and make-up products labeled as non-comedogenic or oil-free.

five. Protect your skin from the solar: Sun publicity can cause hyperpigmentation and make bigger the restoration method for zits scars. Apply a large-spectrum sunscreen with an SPF of 30 or better each day, even on cloudy days, to defend your pores and skin. Wearing a substantial-brimmed hat and looking for coloration whilst possible also can help shield your pores and pores and skin from sun harm.

6. Control irritation: Reducing infection can help prevent zits scars, as inflamed pores and pores and skin is much more likely to result in scarring. Incorporate anti inflammatory skin care elements, which includes niacinamide or inexperienced tea extract, into your routine. Additionally, take into account making manner of existence changes to lessen contamination, which includes keeping a healthful healthy dietweight-reduction plan, dealing with stress, and getting enough sleep.

7. Be affected man or woman with acne treatments: Acne treatments can take time to expose effects, and looking for to hurry the technique can motive pores and pores and skin damage and scarring. Give your zits remedies several weeks to artwork, and have a look at the commands furnished with the useful aid of your dermatologist or skin care professional. If a treatment is not jogging after the great quantity of time,

consult your dermatologist for similarly guidance.

By following those tips and keeping a proactive technique to acne manipulate, you may reduce the risk of growing zits scars and sell more healthy, clearer pores and skin.

Topical Treatments for Scarring:

Topical remedies can be an effective way to decorate the advent of zits scars via selling pores and pores and pores and skin recuperation, reducing discoloration, and stimulating collagen manufacturing. Here are a few extended reasons of topical remedies for scarring:

1. Topical retinoids: Retinoids, which include tretinoin and adapalene, paintings with the beneficial useful resource of growing cell turnover and selling collagen manufacturing, which could help beautify the advent of zits scars. They additionally help in decreasing hyperpigmentation and

night time out skin tone. Consult a dermatologist to determine if a topical retinoid is suitable for your precise goals and to talk about capacity side outcomes, which includes dryness or inflammation.

2. Alpha hydroxy acids (AHAs): AHAs, including glycolic and lactic acid, are chemical exfoliants that assist eliminate useless skin cells, sell mobile turnover, and stimulate collagen manufacturing, enhancing the arrival of zits scars. AHAs may be found in numerous skincare merchandise, which embody cleansers, toners, and serums. Start with a decrease awareness and regularly increase the energy as your skin tolerates the acid. Be cautious whilst the use of AHAs, as they're able to make your pores and pores and skin more touchy to the sun; continuously apply sunscreen for the duration of the day.

three. Vitamin C: Vitamin C is a powerful antioxidant that permits brighten the pores and pores and skin, lessen hyperpigmentation, and enhance the arrival of zits scars. Look for a nutrients C serum or cream with a strong shape of vitamins C, at the facet of ascorbic acid or magnesium ascorbyl phosphate. Vitamin C also can help shield your skin from environmental stressors, which encompass pollution and UV damage.

four. Niacinamide: Niacinamide, a form of diet B3, can assist lessen infection, redness, and hyperpigmentation associated with zits scars. This element also lets in supply a boost to the pores and pores and skin's barrier function, making it extra resilient to outside stressors. Niacinamide may be determined in diverse skincare merchandise, inclusive of serums, lotions, and toners.

five. Azelaic acid: Azelaic acid is a obviously taking vicinity acid that would help reduce irritation, hyperpigmentation, and improve pores and skin texture. This element is particularly beneficial for people with darker pores and pores and skin tones who may be extra prone to put up-inflammatory hyperpigmentation. Azelaic acid may be decided in prescription-strength formulations similarly to over the counter products.

6. Peptides: Peptides are brief chains of amino acids that act as constructing blocks for proteins like collagen and elastin, which provide pores and skin its firmness and elasticity. Using peptide-infused pores and skin care merchandise can assist stimulate collagen production, improving the appearance of acne scars. Peptides may be positioned in serums, creams, and special pores and skin care merchandise.

7. Silicone gel: Silicone gel can assist enhance the appearance of raised scars with the beneficial aid of developing a protective barrier on the pores and skin, promoting hydration, and lowering infection. It is generally carried out as a skinny layer over the scarred area and may be located in

severa over-the-counter merchandise, which include gels, sheets, and creams.

Remember that consistency and endurance are key on the equal time as the usage of topical treatments for scarring. It can also take numerous weeks or perhaps months to peer giant enhancements in the appearance of pimples scars. If you're uncertain which treatment is maximum suitable to your specific scarring or pores and pores and skin type, seek advice from a dermatologist or skin care expert for guidance.

Professional Treatments for Acne Scars:

In a few times, expert remedies can be crucial to obtain considerable improvements in the advent of pimples scars. These treatments frequently include superior technology or techniques to stimulate collagen production, take away broken pores and skin layers, and promote skin healing. Here are some extended reasons of professional remedies for acne scars:

1. Chemical peels: Chemical peels contain the software of a chemical technique to the pores and pores and skin to remove the outermost layers and stimulate collagen manufacturing. The energy of the peel determines the depth of exfoliation and the extent of pores and skin development. Mild peels, like glycolic acid, can be carried out by means of using the use of an aesthetician, whilst medium to deep peels, like TCA, want to be completed with the aid of a dermatologist or a professional expert.

2. Microdermabrasion: Microdermabrasion is a non-invasive treatment that gently exfoliates the pores and skin via spraying tiny crystals or the use of a diamond-tipped tool to get rid of the outermost layer of dull pores and skin cells. This machine promotes collagen production and improves the arrival of zits scars.

Multiple periods can be had to gain favored effects, and it's miles exquisite relevant for mild to mild scarring.

3. Microneedling: Microneedling, moreover referred to as collagen induction treatment, involves the usage of a tool with tiny needles to create managed micro-accidents within the pores and pores and skin. This manner stimulates the body's herbal restoration reaction, promoting collagen and elastin manufacturing, which can assist enhance the arrival of zits scars. Microneedling can be blended with platelet-wealthy plasma (PRP) remedy for additonal consequences.

four. Laser treatment: Laser remedy uses targeted moderate electricity to eliminate the affected pores and skin layers, stimulate collagen manufacturing, and enhance the appearance of zits scars. There are diverse styles of laser remedies to be had, along with ablative lasers, non-ablative lasers, and fractional laser resurfacing, every with notable tiers of depth and downtime. A dermatologist can assist determine the most appropriate laser treatment on your unique acne scars and dreams.

five. Dermal fillers: Dermal fillers, which encompass hyaluronic acid fillers or collagen-stimulating fillers, can assist speedy beautify the appearance of atrophic pimples scars via together with amount to the affected regions. Fillers can offer right away results, however they may be no longer a eternal solution, because of the fact the body will progressively take in the filler over time.

6. Subcision: Subcision is a minor surgical remedy that includes the use of a needle or a small scalpel to release fibrous bands underneath the pores and pores and skin that tether scars to the underlying tissue. This technique is specifically useful for rolling scars and can be mixed with different treatments, along with fillers or microneedling, for greater great outcomes.

7. Radiofrequency (RF) treatment: Radiofrequency remedy uses energy waves to warmth the deeper layers of the pores and skin, stimulating collagen manufacturing and enhancing the arrival of pimples scars. This treatment may be executed the usage of non-invasive devices or combined with microneedling for extra competitive effects.

It's critical to consult a dermatologist or skincare expert to decide the most suitable remedy for your particular pimples scars and needs. In many instances, a aggregate of treatments can be encouraged to advantage the splendid outcomes. Keep in thoughts that treating zits scars can take time, and endurance is essential to seeing considerable improvements on your pores and skin's look.

Chapter 7: Understanding Acne

Acne is the most not unusual pores and pores and skin trouble inside the international everybody will ought to address it in the long run and doing so isn't always any amusing in any respect! From the uncomfortable itchiness to the ugly spots, pimples is a pain from start to complete, and it's even extra distressing even as it occurs while you're properly past your teenage years. Of path, you want to eliminate it as rapid as feasible, however before we start talking about remedies; we'll need to take a better take a look at acne so that you could higher understand the manner to treat it.

Most people equate the term "pimples" with pimples. This isn't too a long manner off the mark, however there's a piece bit extra to it than that. The medical definition of zits (and, certain, it is a systematic scenario, make no mistake about that) is that it's what takes place at the same time as your hair follicles or pores get clogged up. These blockages can typically be blamed on a buildup of more oil. This oil, or sebum, is produced via your sebaceous glands and it usually does the undertaking of preserving your pores and pores and pores and skin from drying out. When there's too much of it, however, it makes your pores and pores and skin greasy and traps useless pores and pores and skin cells to your pores – giving microbes an opportunity to invade. These bacteria, in turn, are accountable for the pores and pores and skin lesions associated with zits.

The Causes of Acne

Many factors bring about an excessive production of oil. Most of the time, a terrible case of spots may be blamed for extended degrees of androgens on your tool. This circle of relatives of hormones is responsible for the development of secondary intercourse traits in each women and men, but it additionally causes your sebaceous glands to provide greater oil than is vital. The outbreaks of pimples professional for the duration of puberty for each boys and ladies, and in advance than menstruation in girls, can as a result be blamed on the extent of androgens that normally spike at the ones times. Other motives of zits embody medications that encompass lithium, corticosteroids, androgens, or comparable compounds, similarly to eating excessive-glycemic components and the not unusual use of greasy make-up. The thing to keep in thoughts, however, is that your susceptibility to zits can also be genetic – if participants of your right now own family suffered from zits, it's likely that you may too.

To be extra specific, here is a short evaluation at the possible inner motives of your acne. One is someone's allergic reaction or the overproduction of male hormones referred to as androgens. This hormone is accountable for sebum or oil manufacturing, which lubricates the pores and pores and pores and skin and protects it from out of doors contamination. But do not forget that the micro organism that motive pimples are not foreign places to the human body.

The overproduction of androgens in girls may be because of a number of different factors. These factors embody however aren't limited to; Adrenal Adaptation / Fatigue Syndrome, Insulin Resistance, Polycystic Ovary Syndrome, Pregnancy, Excessive Stress, and Menopause.

If you are a woman laid low with character pimples, then having your hormones checked is probably the number one factor you ought to do in case you want to find out the fastest answer possible. But in case you're each a person or even though in your teenage years, then there's a huge sort of home treatments you could attempt which could in reality repair your pimples problems.

Finally, the pimples situation is attached immediately with the Propionibacterium acnes or P. Acnes micro organism. It is basically the bacteria that flourishes in clogged pores and blocked hair follicles; commonly triggering an inflammatory motion via the individual's immune tool. The inflammation usually persists till the clogged pore is certainly uninterested in the abscesses (oil, vain pores and pores and pores and skin cells, and bacteria) inner it. The final fabricated from this chain of activities is the scary pimples.

Acne Symptoms

Acne commonly takes location on the face and neck, even though it isn't unusual for it to be located at the shoulders, back, and chest as well. Typically, you understand you've were given zits whilst you get pores and skin lesions, or areas wherein the tissue is broken.

Sometimes, a specific spot inside the pores and pores and skin will itch some days in advance than displaying any symptoms and signs of zits. This is why it's miles in no manner satisfactory to scratch your face for any itches as this can unfold the infection to neighboring follicles/pores.

The following types of skin lesions are the primary signs of a case of acne:

Pimples

Pimples are the pores and pores and pores and skin lesions most typically related to pimples. You won't observe whiteheads or blackheads, but the second you discover a zit in your face, alarm bells start to burst off. These emerge at the identical time as a follicle becomes infected to the element in which its walls have already been damaged down, permitting the micro organism and pus to unfold to the surrounding place. If the contamination isn't too bad, you'll get papules, or small, crimson bumps that experience tender and purpose pain while you poke them (or even in case you don't). If there's a buildup of pus, but, you'll get pustules instead, and those are the irritated, red pimples that have white spots of their centers (that white stuff, which comes out if you pop your pimples, is the pus).

Whiteheads

Whiteheads take place when your pores come to be clogged with oil that hasn't reached the pores and pores and skin but. The blockage is positioned decrease down in the thin duct that connects the sebaceous gland to the floor of your pores and skin, and that's why the ones are so difficult to remove. It's lucky that their mild shade makes them distinctly unnoticeable in assessment to the other lesions.

Blackheads

Contrary to well-known belief, blackheads are not due to dirt getting trapped inner your pores. Rather, they're normal whilst vain pores and pores and skin cells and bacteria get trapped on your oil ducts near the floor of your pores and pores and skin. Because they're uncovered to air, the ones blockages get oxidized fairly fast, which in flip gives them their darkish colour.

Nodules

Nodules shape decrease within the pores and skin than blackheads, whiteheads, or pimples, and they may be associated with excessive pimples outbreaks. These are massive, inflamed lumps beneath the pores and pores and pores and skin which might be firm to touch and painful.

Cysts

Cysts are placed in truly lousy instances of zits. Like nodules, those lesions rise up within the deeper layers of the pores and pores and skin, however they're complete of pus and can be wrong for boils. These may be very painful, and could almost surely leave scars and pitting. Neither these nor nodules are without problem treatable the usage of topical remedy.

Chapter 2

Herbal Remedies

Sometimes, going traditional is excellent. These herbal treatments can provide each right now and prolonged-lasting remedy, and loads of them had been used for loads of years. The gadgets in this listing are smooth to advantage and use – in truth, many can be effects located in your own home and kitchen. So, there may be sure to be a few thing for you right here. If you're unsure the manner you'll react (sensitivity-realistic) to any of those, but, don't hesitate to consult your doctor to discover inside the occasion that they're stable for you.

Tea Tree Oil

Tea tree oil is a very popular pimples treatment. In fact, it's integrated into some of lotions and cosmetics simply so they won't be as harsh at the skin as their chemically-based opposite numbers. Scientific studies have even shown that it's far definitely as effective as some over-the-counter acne drugs, so this crucial oil from the Australian outback is a great wager for all people looking for to clear up their spots.

In order to cope with pimples, you need to dab a touch tea tree oil at once for your pimples at the same time as you've wiped smooth your face. It is simple to discover, specifically as an pimples treatment within the form of solutions and creams that may be offered from most drug shops. Just be cautious no longer to swallow any – while tea tree oil is flawlessly safe for topical use, it can cause toxic reactions that range in severity (from rashes to comas) if you ingest it.

Aloe Vera

Aloe Vera is used as a home remedy for such a lot of subjects that it shouldn't come as a wonder that it could be utilized in competition to zits as nicely. It will for this reason be nicely certainly worth your whilst to domesticate this plant, which can be easily grown in a small pot. To put off your spots, all you'll want to do is pluck a clean leaf and squeeze it to get the polysaccharide-rich gel, which you have to then examine to your zits. Let it live there for round five minutes in advance than washing it off with smooth water and permitting your pores and skin to air dry. You can try this each day as long as your zits are nevertheless present.

Lemon Juice

Lemon juice consists of alpha hydroxy acids that go through a setting resemblance to the lively factors of many anti-pimples medicines. It is likewise a natural astringent that might assist get rid of useless pores and pores and skin cells and unclog pores.

The simplest way to use lemon juice as a treatment is to squeeze some fresh lemon and rub the juice for your acne earlier than you fall asleep to provide it time to work. You can then wash it off even as you wake up. Alternatively, you could mixture the lemon juice with an same quantity of rose water to mood its acidity, and use the resulting solution as a slight facial wash. Since lemon juice is an exfoliant, it can make your skin extra at risk of sunburn. So, stay out of the solar for a while after utilizing this treatment. The acidity also can make it sting a chunk, mainly if your zits are virtually infected. If the pain will become an excessive amount of for you, you can try to use apricot juice in a comparable manner.

Grape Seed Extract

Grape seed extract is known to have very powerful disinfectant homes, and it additionally has hundreds of weight-reduction plan E. You can with out issue buy a bottle at your nearest fitness shop. Just disperse 10 to 40 drops of this in half of a cup of water, and use a cotton swab to use this combination to the infected areas.

Cucumber

You've already heard how you may use cucumber to soothe your pores and skin and reduce puffiness round your worn-out eyes, however it is able to do extra than that with regards to skin care. These greens are ninety five% water, this means that that that that they'll assist moisturize your skin and because of this maintain the accumulation of vain pores and skin cells to a minimal. They may additionally even assist clear your pores and cast off masses of extra oil.

Get the most from a remedy via blitzing a peeled cucumber and spreading the subsequent slush in your trouble areas. Wash this off with clean water after a couple of minutes.

Witch Hazel Bark

Witch hazel bark has lengthy been used to deal with zits. It owes its effectiveness to the tannins it incorporates, which make it a natural exfoliant that may dispose of useless pores and skin cells and sell the boom of greater recent, more healthy ones.

To use witch hazel bark in your acne, boil five to ten grams of the bark in a cup of water. Filter out the bark while you've acquired the extract, and use the liquid to clean your face (and other problem areas) to 3 times a day, relying on the severity of your acne. White all rightand English walnut bark can every be used in a comparable manner if you can't search out witch hazel.

Garlic

Aside from its uses in the kitchen, garlic is perception for its antimicrobial and antifungal houses. The calcium, zinc, sulfur, and allicin that it contains make garlic a first rate pores and skin-cleansing agent for those with zits.

Treatment is as smooth as unpeeling a clove of garlic and rubbing it to your pimples severa times an afternoon, with the intention to relieve the pain and itching and to make the lesions dry quicker. Alternatively, you can mixture crushed garlic with water and look at the following paste to infected pores and skin. This may not be the remedy to apply in advance than a heat date, however it's miles surprisingly powerful.

Tomatoes

Tomatoes aren't sincerely healthful eats. The equal homes that reason them to so pinnacle on your healthy eating plan – at the aspect of an abundance of lycopene, and nutrients A, C, and K – also reason them to effective anti-acne entrepreneurs. The herbal acidity of tomatoes additionally makes lesions dry up and, therefore, heal quicker.

You can use this skin-clearing approach by way of the use of really reducing a tomato and setting it at the inflamed regions of your pores and pores and pores and skin. You also can mash multiple tomatoes to apply as a recuperation facial masks.

Potatoes

Potatoes consist of massive quantities of vitamins B and C, which promote pores and skin regeneration from the bottom up and help guard the pores and skin from damage. They also are rich in niacin, so that you can assist lighten the darkish spots that acne often depart of their wake. All you'll need to do is observe raw shredded potato to your problem regions.

Chickpea Flour and Turmeric

Chickpea flour is a gentle exfoliant, which you can turn to if such things as lemon juice and tannins feel too harsh for you. For the pleasant anti-zits effect, it could be combined with floor turmeric, as this spice is a herbal antiseptic and antioxidant. Mix those elements with a bit milk or yogurt to make a paste, which you may then use as a facial mask. Just make sure to go smooth at the turmeric, as an excessive amount of of it is able to deliver your pores and pores and skin a yellow tinge (don't fear, this will wash off subsequently). You may additionally ought to test a hint to get the proportions precisely right for your pores and skin tone.

Basil Herbal Wash

Even while dried, basil leaves have high-quality antimicrobial homes, and they will help combat irritation as properly. So, get organized to raid your spice rack for this treatment! Shake out 2 to 4 teaspoons of dried basil leaves and boil them in a cup of water. Let this combination steep (and cool) for round 20 mins, and use it to easy your face.

Honey

All types of restoration residences are attributed to honey, and for great motive. Raw honey has been mounted to be a big antibacterial agent, and also you pleasant want to take a look at its statistics in traditional and alternative treatment to be happy of the fact. Honey's antibacterial residences with out being too harsh on the pores and skin make it an wonderful choice for a natural purifier. Since honey (Again, Manuka honey is normally advocated) moisturizes your pores and pores and skin with minimum hazard of infection, it may also be used as a day by day cleaner. Since it is stated that there might be a few folks who are allergic to honey, so make sure you carry out an hypersensitivity test in different elements of your pores and pores and skin. Manuka honey from New Zealand, specially, is concept to be powerful in opposition to acne, and it's miles recommended that you smear a small amount of this in your acne, leaving it to sit overnight, over the path of a few days.

The honey you could buy domestically can art work sincerely as well, however. Try blending it with a bit of cinnamon bark (that is an anti-inflammatory agent) to create a harm-repairing facial masks. Refer to Chapter 6 for extra information approximately the way to create and use selfmade facemasks.

Chapter three

Anti-Acne Diet

Acne isn't in simple terms an out of doors scenario – internal imbalances also can make a contribution to the severity of a virulent disease. You may not be able to do a good deal about your hormones (puberty and menstruation are natural stages in existence, and hormone substitute remedy will quality be advocated for the maximum extreme instances), but you may manipulate what you eat. Yes, your food plan can play a huge feature in pimples treatment and prevention. In this bankruptcy, we'll communicate about the meals you need to eat and people you ought to avoid so as to benefit extra healthy pores and skin.

What to Eat

For the maximum factor, the anti-pimples diet plan is surely healthy consuming – it pleasant makes experience that wholesome meals will reason healthy skin. Still, you may likely want some help on that factor, so this listing enumerates what you need to stock up on in case you want to overcome a case of zits.

Alfalfa

These nutrient-rich sprouts can do wonders for assisting preserve your pores and skin clean. Since you could get them very glowing (you may buy developing alfalfa sprouts even in supermarkets), they may but include stay anti inflammatory enzymes by the point they make their manner onto your plate.

Artichoke

Artichokes are chock complete of weight loss plan C and antioxidants, which makes them outstanding for clearing your frame of free radicals that would inhibit the renewal of your pores and pores and skin.

Beets

The juice of beetroots can be used to stimulate your liver a outstanding way to assist hasten the degradation and elimination of pollutants to your frame. For the high-quality effect, integrate one part beet juice with three factors carrot juice and additives water to make a cleansing drink.

Broccoli

Since your susceptibility to zits can be irritated through way of loose radicals to your machine, the anti-oxidant-wealthy broccoli will bypass an extended way closer to making your pores and skin blemish unfastened. Just make sure now not to overcook this vegetable, as on the way to lower the effectiveness of the nutrients A, B complex, C, E, and K that broccoli contains.

Coriander and Cumin

Coriander and cumin are every anti inflammatory and antibacterial shops which can be regularly used in Ayurvedic remedy. You might also want to make a tasty herbal tea thru blending half of a teaspoon every of cumin, coriander, and fennel, and letting them steep in warm water for as a minimum 10 minutes.

Fennel

Fennel root will help reduce more fluids and pollution for your pores and skin. In addition to that, it lets in decorate your digestion and is pretty tasty as nicely (the taste is harking back to licorice).

Fish

Fatty fish like salmon, mackerel, tuna, and herring are rich in vital fatty acids which include omega-three and omega-6. These are very powerful in combating contamination and lowering the redness round acne lesions.

Fresh Fruits

There are such a lot of end result that you could consume to assist fight pimples. Different end result consist of pretty a few antioxidants, vitamins, and anti inflammatory compounds, and provide a massive kind of tastes and textures that permits you to enchantment to any palate. Good alternatives to comprise into your anti-acne food plan embody apples, apricots, avocados, bananas, bilberries, cantaloupes, cherries, figs, red grapes, mangoes, papaya, and passion fruit.

Nuts

Most varieties of nuts additionally include anti-inflammatory omega-three fatty acids. They additionally have minerals no longer quite virtually positioned in masses of diverse components, which includes zinc, selenium, copper, magnesium, potassium, and iron, deficiencies of which can be associated with acne outbreaks.

Whole Grains

Whole grains are rich in fiber, as a manner to assist flush volatile fats and pollutants out of your digestive tract in advance than they have got a threat to gather your pores and pores and skin. Many grains (like brown rice) furthermore comprise weight-reduction plan B, which permits you fight acne-causing stress as properly.

Vitex

Vitex is slightly greater extraordinary than maximum of these options, however it can be well without a doubt properly well worth the little bit of extra attempt that it will take to get keep of it. The fruit of this plant, which is likewise known as the chasteberry, has been used to deal with the zits outbreaks associated with women's durations for the purpose that time of the ancient Greeks and Romans. You'll ought to use the complete fruit for this, which you may get inside the shape of dried berries. These are unpalatably bitter, so that you can also need to take them inside the form of a tincture combined with particular herbs to decorate the flavor.

What to Avoid

There are also food which can worsen your acne in case you consume an excessive amount of of them, so it's superb to avoid them or lessen them from your diet absolutely while you're looking for to combat off a lousy case of spots. These encompass the following:

Trans-fat and saturated fat

It only makes revel in that eating greasy meals will give you greasy pores and pores and skin, so that you should lessen down on fried subjects and fatty meats. Trans-fats and saturated fats particularly want to be avoided as masses as viable, as your frame could have a extra tough time processing the ones.

Superfluous sugars

Consuming foods and drinks that embody excessive quantities of sugar can cause an increase for your body's insulin levels, which in turn stimulates the manufacturing of androgens – this could simply make breakouts worse. So, to your next run for groceries, try and face up to choosing up sodas, sweetened juices, chocolates, and baked items.

Excess carbohydrates

Starchy food that include a number of processed carbohydrates can motive pretty lots the equal acne-inducing conditions as meals which have loads of sugar. If you've gotten used to having white bread for breakfast and snacking on potato chips, look for whole-grain or legume-based totally completely alternatives (which encompass whole wheat bread and roasted peanuts).

Spicy foods

Spicy meals and warm peppers can once in a while bring about terrible instances of acne rosacea, in which redness suffuses the pores and skin in hassle areas – and that takes location in addition to the zits. That's a quite proper purpose to maintain the chili and ethnic food on maintain.

Dairy merchandise

Milk and special dairy merchandise like cheese, cream, or perhaps ice cream include hormones which could stimulate your sebaceous glands to growth oil manufacturing. If you can't circulate with out milk, go with soy- or almond-based virtually merchandise as an alternative.

Salt

It has been positioned that multiplied iodine ranges regularly accompany bad instances of zits. For this reason, it's an fantastic concept to cut down on salt and salty meals, collectively with canned meats and maximum kinds of chips, no matter whether or not or no longer or now not they are fabricated from potatoes or corn flour.

Certain stop result and greens

Some stop end result and vegetables can cause imbalances in your pores and pores and skin's pH which could cause the proliferation of micro organism there. To hold this from happening, limit your intake of squash, pumpkin, lentils, plums, corn, cranberries, and currants.

Chapter four

Lifestyle Changes to Beat Acne

Even with the right varieties of treatment and weight loss program, you will despite the fact that want to make some adjustments in your manner of existence on the way to virtually beat acne. In this financial disaster, we listing some behaviors that you have to turn out to be conduct, so you will constantly be one step in advance on the subject of controlling a case of zits.

Wash Problem Areas, But Don't Go Overboard

The first thriller to beating pimples is to maintain your face and one of a kind hassle areas easy. Make nice to scrub as a minimum two times an afternoon, and in no way doze off with a dirty face. Women, especially, need to make an effort to get rid of all lines of makeup in advance than going to bed. The extremely good way to clean your trouble areas is to wash them with lukewarm water and a slight purifier, the usage of your hands or a moderate cloth. Don't make a dependancy of scrubbing too tough or the usage of an exfoliating product as your ordinary cleanser – doing this could aggravate your pores and pores and skin and purpose infection, making you even more susceptible to acne. You ought to additionally keep away from the temptation to scrub your face continuously, due to the truth that, contrary to famous belief, this could virtually dry out your pores and pores and skin and now not assist in any respect.

Common feel also dictates that specific hygiene includes making sure that any items your bring in contact collectively in conjunction with your acne-susceptible regions have to be clean as well. Don't overuse the flannel you operate for laundry your face, and alternate the towels you use to dry off afterwards at least as quickly as in step with week. Launder those devices thoroughly, and store them in a clean, dry cabinet or cupboard. It will also be beneficial to smooth makeup brushes in heat soapy water at least as soon as every month, and to throw out sponges and applicators which have seen an excessive amount of use.

Clean Hair Means Clear Skin

If you're suffering from an zits outbreak, you need to make greater try and keep your hair easy. This is due to the truth your hair can lure germs and dust, and it is all too easy for the ones to get transferred from there for your face, shoulders, and neck. Wash your hair regularly, and don't watch for it to get all lank and greasy, in particular if it's lengthy sufficient to cling down your decrease lower back. It is likewise a splendid idea to save you the use of things like gels, oily go away-on products and pomades, due to the fact the grease from these can make a contribution to the clogging of your pores.

If you're looking to fight off a intense case of acne, maintain your hair up and hold it away from your face in the interim. It may also help in case you sleep with it contained in a hair net or caught up in a braid, to preserve your self from rubbing your face toward it at some level within the night. If topics are simply awful, it might be first-class if you'd get a lessen with the intention to absolutely hold your hair off your lower once more, shoulders, and face.

Ease Up on the Makeup

Minimize your use of makeup, due to the fact each greater problem that you smear for your face can contribute in your acne problem. Cream and liquid merchandise specially have a dependancy of operating their way into pores. If you may't do without makeup, use powdered products rather (though exercise them sparingly even though).

You need to additionally keep away from setting onto your cosmetics for too lengthy. Bacteria can begin to boom in such harmless places as your mascara or your lipstick, so if you've were given some issue more than a three hundred and sixty five days vintage, throw it out.

Learn to Control Stress

High stages of sustained strain can bring about acne outbreaks, or get worse the condition in case you already have it. Try your first-rate to keep away from conditions which you realise will strain you out, and if you may't get out of them (you obtained't be able to genuinely ditch college or paintings, for instance), have a take a look at strategies to control your response to them. Alleviating pressure can be as smooth as talking for your friends and own family, or sincerely giving your self a weekly deal with, like a movie or an brilliant dinner, so you'll have a few element to look in advance to whilst you get beyond some thing's causing you strain. Regular exercise, healthy sound asleep conduct, and calming techniques (like meditation and deep respiration) can even help.

Don't Pop Your Zits!

The constant touching of zits-inflamed pores and skin and, worse, the pricking or popping of pimples will not help in any respect. This will remarkable go together with the go with the flow dirt and micro organism from your palms onto your pores and skin and, in the case of popping, unfold the bacteria-stuffed pus round, making your even extra vulnerable to contamination! Ignore the urge to scratch, poke, and prick the least bit costs. It may additionally help to preserve a pressure ball on your pocket or purse, so that you can reap for that as an alternative every time you sense tempted.

Change Your Pillowcases!

A hassle that sometimes leads to zits breakouts is the dust and oil left over to your pillowcases as you sleep. This hassle is more observable in folks that sleep with their faces in competition to their pillows. To prevent this trouble from inflicting your zits, attempt to make it a dependancy to exchange your pillowcases as a minimum 2-3 times each week.

Chapter 5

Over-the-counter Acne Products

There isn't always any denying that herbal treatments and remedies for zits may be very effective and are showed with hundreds of fulfillment. But don't forget that treating pimples the usage of herbal remedies can take severa weeks to expose results. If you omit out on any brilliant enhancements for your pores and skin after eight-10 weeks, you need to strive a top notch herbal remedy or you may strive over-the-counter zits products.

While a few pimples remedies and tablets can be very luxurious, low cost pimples products which incorporates Benzoyl Peroxide creams or gels are available in most drugstores and even supermarkets. Just recall that some humans may moreover have allergies with fantastic over-the-counter acne merchandise. Although those instances may be as an alternative unusual, you have to continuously test and do your very personal research at the same time as utilizing or eating acne drug treatments. The same diploma of caution want to additionally be positioned with the aid of manner of human beings who've very sensitive pores and pores and skin.

To come up with an define of those over-the-counter zits drug treatments, here is a listing of the pinnacle treatments with the maximum opinions of fulfillment:

Benzoyl Peroxide

Benzoyl peroxide (or what others talk to as BP) is a totally well-known over the counter treatment for zits. It is a topical medicine that usually comes in creams, lotions, gels, soaps, and incredible liquids that may be applied right away on the skin.

Benzoyl peroxide dissolves any blockages within the pores and is formulated to kill zits-inflicting micro organism (P. Acnes) and save you them from spreading.

A drawback to using benzoyl peroxide to deal with your pimples is that it commonly has a purging length wherein the circumstance in quick receives worse first. This is due to the fact the medicine is attempting to cleanse from deep inside the pores and pores and skin and combat the pimples-inflicting micro organism. This commonly takes location in the course of the second to 4th week upon beginning the treatment.

During this time period, some of aspect results also can occur. These not unusual aspect results embody but are not limited to; excessively dry pores and pores and pores and skin, peeling pores and skin, warmth pores and pores and skin, and tingling/stinging pores and pores and skin.

As you could already recognize, benzoyl peroxide isn't always andovernight' remedy for acne. This technique it can absorb to four-6 weeks earlier than your pimples indicates crucial improvements. This is because of the reality benzoyl peroxide is formulated as a permanent and extended-term answer, and targets to deal with particularly mild to severe acne.

Products that comprise benzoyl peroxide are available strengths starting from 2.5% to ten%. To be steady, begin with a product with only 2.Five% benzoyl peroxide to look if the product is clearly too harsh to your pores and pores and skin.

Salicylic Acid

Salicylic acid is taken into consideration as the second maximum famous over the counter pimples product subsequent to benzoyl peroxide. It is certainly an energetic thing for quite some face washes, face creams, and exceptional pores and pores and pores and skin cleansers.

The motion of salicylic acid efficiently dries up pimples which include whiteheads and blackheads. It additionally stimulates the cellular turnover price. This hastens the dropping of dead skin cells, which can be fundamental while your pores and pores and skin starts offevolved to peel.

Salicylic acid merchandise are available in pads, cleansers, and every now and then lotions and creams. A large factor impact of the usage of salicylic acid is pores and skin redness, this is from time to time followed via manner of slight tingling and dryness. This is a ordinary reaction and have to no longer be the motive for panic. If the redness or dryness deems an excessive amount of for you, you could lessen your use of the product and adjust for your comfort stage.

Retinoid

Using topical retinoid to cope with acne is likewise a famous choice for humans laid low with zits. It can be used for optimum all severity levels — but is wonderful at the identical time as used with a product that kills zits-causing micro organism which include benzoyl peroxide.

The use of topical retinoids is one of the next stuff you want to try if your zits fails to reply to one in all a kind remedies. This works because of the fact the movement of retinoids is to unclog pores through the use of the use of normalizing hyperkeratinization – a illness wherein useless pores and skin cells internal a hair follicle is avoided from being sloughed off due to the overproduction of keratin which plugs the follicle and leads to acne breakouts. Retinoids also are said to have effective anti-inflammatory outcomes, which lessen the redness and swelling of a pimple.

Retinoids can take a totally long term (spherical 3 to 6 months) in advance than results start to show. Also bear in thoughts that retinoids might not be as effective through manner of way of itself as at the same time as combined with each different topical product.

Antibiotics

There is likewise some of extremely good antibiotics that could every be used orally or topically to kill zits-causing micro organism. Although some antibiotic medications for acne require a medical doctor's prescription, there are a few over-the-counter topical antibiotics that can powerful kill zits-causing micro organism.

A famous antibiotic for treating zits is clindamycin. Topical clindamycin is to be had in gels, creams, and special drinks. Clindamycin is probably very powerful a number of bacterial infections (which include P. Acnes). It actively kills those micro organism and forestalls their growth. Another famous antibiotic for pimples is doxycycline. It is used for treating extreme acne with large fulfillment rate.

A challenge with the usage of antibiotics to cope with pimples is the 'antibiotic resistance' of the P. Acnes. This typically takes place with the extended use of a particular antibiotic on the pores and pores and skin. This is why it is important not to use a particular antibiotic to cope with zits for extra than a yr.

Precautions at the same time as the use of over-the-counter acne merchandise

The first trouble you need to consider is that those treatments can also require a massive quantity of time earlier than observable consequences. During remedy, it's far vital no longer to use too many anti-acne merchandise at any given term besides for topical retinoids. Applying an excessive amount of merchandise may also moreover purpose infection, which in addition aggravates the situation – fundamental to excessive redness, flakiness, and occasionally pain and puffiness in the pores and pores and skin. Also, it is important to prevent using an zits product at the same time as your pores and skin begins offevolved itching or displaying different signs and symptoms which encompass blisters, swelling, burning sensation, rashes, chronic redness, and once in a while fever.

Using Moisturizers

A way to lessen the issue effects of maximum of the anti-acne merchandise above is to use a moisturizer to fight immoderate dryness of the pores and pores and skin. As the decision indicates, moisturizers are topical merchandise which might be used to hold the hydration and moisture of the ground of your pores and pores and skin. Some moisturizers have sun safety element or SPF which protects your pores and pores and skin from the UV rays of the solar. This is particularly powerful in stopping publish-inflammatory hyperpigmentation or PIH – the darkish marks or spots left over from an acne infection. Information on the way to lessen publish-inflammatory hyperpigmentation is probably cited next financial destroy.

When choosing a moisturizer to use on your pores and skin, hold in thoughts to test if it's miles labeled as 'non-comedogenic' and oil-loose. This is due to the fact a few moisturizers can block pores, which can also bring about a breakout.

Finally, using moisturizers is proper best for humans with dry pores and pores and pores and skin or with peeling pores and skin. People with manifestly oily pores and pores and skin have already got extra than enough moisture on their pores and skin. Applying moisturizer while you have got already were given an oily pores and skin will only make it worse. But you can despite the truth that need pores and pores and skin protection from the sun so that you also can need to use a non-comedogenic sunscreen as an alternative.

Prescription Medication for Acne

It is not any secret that prescription medication and professional remedies on your acne can be luxurious. It is normally advocated handiest as a very last lodge while all exclusive domestic treatments have failed.

A famous prescription medication for zits is Accutane (Isotretinoin). It is a prescription drug this is best given for humans with excessive / cystic acne. It straight away combats pimples and its symptoms with the aid of the use of restricting or controlling the sebum production in a affected character's body.

However, destructive effects of taking the drug are pretty common. Since Isotretinoin can be pricey, it is advocated which you take it with caution. Be more cautious in taking Isotretinoin if you have one or more of the subsequent situations: heart ailment, bone sicknesses (osteoporosis, scoliosis, and so on.), illnesses in the intestinal tract, bronchial allergic reactions, diabetes, intellectual illnesses, liver sicknesses, immoderate cholesterol, and eating issues. Finally, isotretinoin ought to by no means be taken by using pregnant women.

An Advice for Using Acne Products

First of all, you have to in no way purchase into 'miracle' remedies that promise quick outcomes. It may be effective for the occasional acne you get right right right here and there. But for real pimples, they're NOT. Remember not to use too many merchandise on your face on the equal time – facial washes that declare to have anti-pimples houses are frequently vain! Stick to the use of a selected remedy and wash your face for a maximum of two times an afternoon using simplest easy water and mild cleaning cleaning cleaning soap.

Finally, you could first use steam to open your pores in advance than using any zits product of face mask (see subsequent financial ruin). To do this, boil about 2-4 cups of smooth water. Make top notch your face is apparent of any makeup and dirt. Transfer the boiled water proper proper right into a smaller subject and drift your head over it. Cover your self with a huge towel to maximise the impact of the steam. Do no longer go along with the flow your face too close to the water because of the fact that it can be very painful! Sit though for approximately 10 mins and pat your face dry.

Chapter 6

Creating Homemade Face Masks for Acne

There is a number of face mask you may create using wonderful materials you may find at domestic. Some face masks have antibacterial houses, moisturizing effects, exfoliating movement, and particular benefits that might assist enhance your pimples.

There are a few materials which can be not unusual for developing face mask that may help enhance your acne. Some have been already mentioned inside the preceding chapters. But this time, their benefits while used as a face mask is probably noted.

First, right here are the maximum well-known substances for developing an acne face masks:

Honey

Besides being beneficial in your fitness and pores and skin on the same time as eaten, honey additionally may be completed without delay on your pores and pores and skin. It also can sound a hint stupid, but honey in reality has very powerful antibacterial homes in addition to soothing and moisturizing consequences. As said in advance, the best sort of honey for use to your face is Manuka honey. You can also moreover want to have a bottle of these as a part of your routine.

Baking Soda

Baking soda is a famous home remedy for treating severa superficial pores and skin situations. It is also known as sodium bicarbonate. It has effective antibacterial homes in addition to exfoliating results that would enhance your pimples. However, uncooked baking soda can be too harsh to the pores and pores and skin whilst used without first diluting it in water or unique beverages. It could be very sturdy in stripping away vain pores and skin cells in addition to stopping pimples-causing micro organism from multiplying.

Lemon Juice

It is already stated earlier how powerful lemon juice is for disinfecting and exfoliating your pores and pores and skin further to lightening pimples marks. Other than definitely rubbing it to your skin to address pimples, it is also a totally famous factor for numerous face mask.

Oatmeal

Aside from being definitely delicious even as cooked and eaten, oatmeal – specially cooked oatmeal – have recovery effects and different blessings even as finished to the skin. Oatmeal efficaciously absorbs and gets rid of gathered oil and micro organism for your pores and skin. It additionally leaves your pores and skin feeling moisturized and smooth after using on your pores and skin.

Egg Whites

Egg whites are very powerful in soaking up extra oil and are very essential for developing pretty a few face mask. This is because the egg whites feature as glue that maintain the factors together similarly to to paste the masks in your pores and pores and skin. Egg whites are especially effective in eliminating whiteheads and blackheads. The protein inside the egg additionally improves the overall situation of your pores and pores and skin. Egg whites even have a pores and skin tightening effect that reduces the arrival of first-rate strains and wrinkles – state-of-the-art improving severa pores and pores and pores and skin conditions on the face.

Apple Cider Vinegar

Apple cider vinegar is a made from fermenting pulverized apples. It is honestly a completely well-known product that has an entire lot of terrific uses collectively with cleansing, food, and as a treatment for a completely big kind of health ailments. Apple cider vinegar is a source of beta-carotene which effectively combats the awful consequences of free radicals. It moreover has antibacterial houses and normalizes hormone imbalance – which might be very beneficial for treating pimples.

The components listed above are number one elements for developing face mask that would cope with your zits. This is because of the fact they'll be effective enough on their personal to provide huge results for your pores and pores and skin. Just go through in mind to apply them with warning mainly baking soda and apple cider vinegar. They can be too much for people with sensitive pores and pores and skin.

The following may be recipes that could consist of one or extra of the foremost factors listed above.

Pure Oatmeal Mask

Oatmeal can be very powerful to be utilized by itself as a face masks. The slight nature of oatmeal additionally makes it best for use daily without worrying approximately an excessive amount of contamination. First, put together dinner one serving of oatmeal the identical manner you would prepare it for ingesting. Allow the oatmeal to sit back off before you have a look at it for your face. You also can use it on the identical time as it's far warmth but snug enough on the same time as left on your face. Make certain you've got got completed a consistency a good way to permit the oatmeal to paste on your face like a masks. For utility, honestly use your hands to apply the oatmeal at the affected regions and leave it on for extra than 10 minutes however never over 15 minutes. Rinse properly with cool water.

Honey Oatmeal Mask

Honey is going mainly properly with the oatmeal masks described above. Oatmeal with honey moreover makes a scrumptious meal this is real authentic in your health as well. So undergo in mind now not to eat the most effective you will be using to your mask. This recipe blessings from the antibacterial houses of the honey. Simply upload approximately 2 tablespoons of honey to the oatmeal and depart for your face for 10-15 mins.

Honey Lemon Face Mask

Lemon's whitening and cleaning residences is the correct mixture for honey's soothing and antibacterial houses. To do that, simply squeeze ½ of the lemon in a bowl and mix it with 1 tbsp. Raw honey. Mix nicely with a spoon and follow on affected regions. This can get a hint messy so it's remarkable finished with a towel nearby to wipe off components that may go in your eyes, all of the manner all of the way right down to your neck, or in your nostril. Leave the mixture on for at least 15 mins or half-hour relying in your loose time. It can be very uncomfortable to move round with this mask on for the purpose that honey can drip right all the manner down to your garments. Rinse nicely with bloodless water and pat dry with a easy towel.

Lemon Egg Face Mask

This face masks recipe is particularly effective for humans with oily pores and pores and skin. Since the egg whites effectively receives rid of oils caught within the pores, the whitening and cleansing impact of lemon juice works plenty higher.

First, you ought to separate the egg white from the yellow yolk. There are many easy techniques you could do to interrupt up the yolk, but the excellent approach is to use an empty water bottle to 'vacuum' the yolk from the egg.

First, positioned the egg on a clean field. Remove the cap of the empty water bottle and squeeze it slightly on the perimeters. Point the mouth of the bottle towards the yolk and launch your squeeze from the bottle. The dashing air ought to suck the yolk inside the bottle even as leaving the egg white within the container.

To create the masks, beat the egg white until it turns frothy. Add within the juice from half of a lemon and blend well. Using your palms, practice and unfold flippantly at the oily factors of your face. Allow the mask to 'settle' and leave it on for round half-hour. Rinse well with water and pat dry with a clean towel. Afterwards, you could have a look at some honey to head lower back the moisture to your pores and skin. To do that, use the records provided on the following recipe.

Baking Soda Mask & Honey Combo

The baking soda mask and honey can be very powerful as a aggregate. However, it's far endorsed that you use them on your face in advance than you visit mattress at night time time.

Baking soda may be used as a slight exfoliating agent with powerful antibacterial residences. To create a clean baking soda masks, add 1-2 tablespoons of baking soda in a small bowl or container. Very slowly; upload small quantities of lukewarm water while stirring along with your palms until the mixture turns into pasty and sticky. Try to use formerly boiled water to make sure it's miles easy. Once finished, observe the masks on hassle regions using round movement. Make positive to spread it lightly in affected regions. DO NOT comply with it too thickly in a specific spot as it could motive inflammation and redness. Wait for the aggregate to grow to be dry and leave it on for best about 5-15 minutes or until the mask turns into hardened. Rinse off with water and pat dry. The baking soda mask is regular to use for fine about instances in line with week. Use it too much and it may over-dry your pores and skin which aggravates pimples.

You can also experience like your pores and skin has tightened significantly after the usage of the baking soda masks. This is because the mask neutralizes any pH imbalances at the skin at the same time as doing away with extra oil that could later grow to be blackheads or whiteheads. However, it's miles crucial which you moisturize right away after the usage of baking soda as a face mask. The first rate moisturizer as of this issue is raw honey. As said in advance in, honey is powerful to be left to your face even in a single day. But this is not vital after using baking soda mask. Just have a look at raw honey on the regions you've used the mask on and leave it on for at the least 1/2-hour. This need to be sufficient to hold your pores and pores and skin moisturized and clean after exfoliating with the baking soda mask.

Honey and Apple Cider Vinegar Mask

Next is the apple cider vinegar with honey face masks. This particular mask is strong in recovery pores and pores and skin lesions, moisturizing overly dry pores and pores and skin, and balancing the pH levels of the pores and skin. This makes it an powerful face mask for human beings with zits-prone pores and skin. To create this face masks, genuinely mix 2 tbsp. Of raw honey and 1 tbsp. Of apple cider vinegar. Apply gently in your face on the identical time as specializing in hassle areas. Leave the mask on for 20-30 minutes earlier than rinsing off with cold water. Again, the honey combination can be very messy to move away in your face. Have a smooth towel or any material prepared to clean drips and one among a type styles of mess.

White Toothpaste

First of all, this does not paintings for gel toothpastes. While now not constantly a 'face mask', occasionally a dab of toothpaste can be an effective spot-treatment for pimples. Using white toothpaste is tested to dry-up zits in a unmarried day. However, this technique nice works best for people with oily pores and pores and skin mainly to people who awaken with oily pores and pores and skin in the morning. This ought to moreover not be implemented for cysts or nodules for the purpose that toothpaste superb dries the topmost layer of your pores and pores and skin. Toothpaste want to moreover now not be used for human beings with very sensitive pores and pores and skin because of the reality the drying effect may also purpose too much dryness which can also worsen the state of affairs. To use toothpaste in treating pimples, located a very small amount in your fingertips and rub lightly on pustules, whiteheads, and blackheads. You can leave it on in a single day and wash it off within the morning.

Obviously, you shouldn't strive the usage of too many face masks at any given time (aside from herbal honey). Abrasive face mask just like the one with baking soda may be too drying to your pores and pores and skin – making it extra touchy even as making use of different topical treatments inclusive of different face mask.

The trick is to find out what precise mask works well together together along with your pores and pores and skin. Just like even as attempting pimples medicine, attempt those masks one by one for at least 2 weeks and note which one produces the pleasant consequences.

Chapter 8: Acne in Maturity

Why me, an man or woman?

Some adults often ask "I'm now not a teenager any further, for what motive do I simply have pores and pores and skin break out?!"

In all fact, it's far very considered ordinary to appearance pores and skin escape keep into maturity. In spite of the reality that pores and skin escape is regularly taken into consideration an trouble of immaturity, it is able to appear in humans, the whole thing being same. Adult zits have numerous likenesses to juvenile pores and pores and pores and skin break out regarding the two motives (hormonal and bacterial) and capsules. Yet, there are a few novel tendencies to grown-up pores and pores and skin infection too.

The four factors that straightforwardly add to pores and skin irritation are: overabundance oil advent pores becoming stopped up by means of using "cheesy" pores and pores and skin cells, microscopic organisms, and aggravation.

There are furthermore a few roundabout elements that effect the previously cited direct factors, which include chemicals, stress, and the monthly cycle in women, all of that may affect oil introduction hair objects, pores and pores and skin health manage devices, and cosmetics, that could save you up pores food plan, which can impact inflammation eventually of the frame. A few prescriptions, which incorporates corticosteroids, anabolic steroids, and lithium, can likewise purpose pores and skin inflammation. Many pores and pores and skin issues, consisting of skin contamination, can be a window right proper into a fundamental state of affairs. For example, going bald, overabundance hair improvement, unpredictable month-to-month cycles, or fast weight gain or misfortune however pores and pores and pores and skin get away, or short beginning of pores and pores and pores and skin get away without a in advance statistics of skin contamination, can be typically warnings of a primary infection, for example, polycystic ovarian scenario, or special endocrine issues.

What reasons man or woman pores and pores and skin infection?

Grown-up pores and skin contamination, or publish-younger man or woman pores and pores and skin infection, is pores and pores and skin infection that takes vicinity after age 25. Generally, the very considers that motive skin break out teenagers are having an effect on the entirety in grown-up pores and pores and skin irritation. The four factors that straightforwardly add to pores and pores and skin inflammation are: overabundance oil advent, pores becoming stopped up via up by "tacky" pores and pores and skin cells, microscopic organisms, and aggravation.

There are moreover some roundabout factors that impact the formerly noted direct factors, which incorporates chemical substances, stress, and the month-to-month cycle in girls, all of that may impact oil creation hair devices, pores and skin fitness control objects, and cosmetics, which could prevent up pores weight loss program, which could effect inflammation for the duration of the body. A few prescriptions, which include corticosteroids, anabolic steroids, and lithium, can likewise purpose pores and pores and skin infection. Many pores and pores and pores and skin troubles, which incorporates pores and pores and skin inflammation, can be a window into a critical condition. For instance, going bald, overabundance hair development, unpredictable monthly cycles, or fast weight advantage or misfortune however pores and pores and skin break out, or short starting of pores and skin get away without a earlier records of pores and pores and skin infection, can be normally warnings of a number one contamination, for instance, polycystic ovarian condition, or distinctive endocrine troubles.

How ought to probable I forestall pimples?

Like maximum topics throughout everyday lifestyles, pores and pores and pores and skin break out isn't always usually absolutely in a single's manipulate. There are, however, some key to assist with forestalling breakouts:

1. Never hit the hay with cosmetics on.

2. Actually have a look at marks: on the same time as looking for corrective and pores and pores and skin care objects, constantly search for the expressions "non-comedogenic," "without oil," or "may not hinder pores."

three. Stay an extended manner from facial oils and hair items that comprise oil. Some acne spots are not in fact pimples however are put up-provocative colour modifications from past pores and pores and skin contamination sores or from deciding on at pores and pores and skin irritation or pimples. Wear sunscreen with SPF 30+ ordinary, a few element may also take region, to stop obscuring of those spots.

Chapter 9: My Zits

How genuinely does rely quantity energy have an effect on the pores and skin?

One problem that might have an impact in your pores and skin is weight loss plan. Certain food property decorate your glucose extra hastily than others. At the point while your glucose rises swiftly, it makes the body discharge insulin-like development thing 1 (IGF-1), a chemical that offers with the affects of development. Having overabundance IGF-1 in your blood could make your oil organs produce greater sebum, growing your dangers of pores and pores and pores and skin escape and contamination.

A few food resources that motive spikes in glucose embody: pasta, white rice, white bread and sugar.

These food kinds are notion of "excessive-glycemic" sugars. That implies they are made from straightforward sugars.

Chocolate is moreover normal to demolish pores and skin escape, but there is not enough superb exploration available to confirm this.

Different scientists have centered on the establishments between a meant "Western diet" or "significant American ingesting habitual" and pores and pores and skin break out. This form of eating regimen relies upon vigorously on: high-glycemic carbs, dairy, soaked fat, trans fat.

These forms of food sources have been located to animate the improvement of chemical materials that could make abundance oil be made and discharged via the use of oil organs. They've likewise found that a Western consuming everyday is connected to extra noteworthy contamination, that would likewise upload to skin get away issues.

What meals assets are common to assist your pores and skin?

Eating low-glycemic meals kinds manufactured from complex starches might also lower your gamble of creating pores and pores and skin break out. Complex starches are tracked down inside the accompanying food kinds: whole grains, vegetables, herbal leafy food.

Food resources containing the accompanying fixings are furthermore remembered to be useful for the skin are:

the mineral zinc, vitamins An and E, synthetics called mobile reinforcements.

Some pores and pores and pores and skin-accommodating food alternatives include:

1. Yellow and orange merchandise of the soil like carrots, apricots, and yams

2. Spinach and one-of-a-type silly inexperienced and verdant greens

3. Tomatoes

four. Blueberries

5. Entire wheat bread

6. Earthy coloured rice

7. Quinoa

eight. Turkey

nine. Pumpkin seeds

10. Beans, peas, and lentils

11. Salmon, mackerel, and one in each of a type sorts of greasy

fishnuts.

Everybody's body is specific, and positive human beings find out that they get extra pores and skin contamination once they eat specific meals kinds. Under your PCP's control, it very well may be useful to find out exceptional avenues regarding your weight loss plan to look what seems extraordinary for you. Continuously don't forget any food sensitivities or awarenesses you would possibly have while arranging your food regimen.

Do any investigations display that those meals kinds assist your pores and skin?

Low-glycemic counts energy

A few overdue examinations recommend that following a low-glycemic healthy dietweight-reduction plan, or one this is low in honest sugars, can prevent and similarly growth pores and pores and skin get away. Specialists in a 2012 take a look at Trusted Wellspring of Korean sufferers determined that following a low-glycemic food regimen for a long term can activate large upgrades in pores and skin get away.

In a modern-day record allotted within the Diary of the American Foundation of Dermatology Trusted Source, scientists located that following a low-glycemic, immoderate-protein diet for a enormous time body in addition developed pores and pores and pores and skin escape in guys, and furthermore brought approximately weight reduction. More modern-day investigations are expected to verify the ones discoveries.

Zinc

Concentrates likewise suggest that eating meals kinds wealthy in zinc might be precious in forestalling and treating pores and pores and skin break out. Food kinds which is probably rich in zinc embody: pumpkin seeds, cashews, hamburger, turkey, quinoa, lentils, fish like shellfish and crab.

www.ingramcontent.com/pod-product-compliance
Lightning Source LLC
Chambersburg PA
CBHW071439080526
44587CB00014B/1912